INVOLVING PATIENTS AND THE PUBLIC

How to do it better

Ruth Chambers

General Practitioner
Professor of Health Commissioning
Staffordshire University

RADCLIFFE MEDICAL PRESS

© 2000 Ruth Chambers

Illustrations © 2000 Martin Davies

Radcliffe Medical Press Ltd
18 Marcham Road, Abingdon, Oxon OX14 1AA

British Library Cataloguing in Publication Data

A catalogue record for this book is available from the British Library.

ISBN 1 85775 393 3

Typeset by Advance Typesetting Ltd, Oxon
Printed and bound by TJ International Ltd, Padstow, Cornwall

► CONTENTS

► ABOUT THE AUTHOR

Ruth Chambers has been a general practitioner for 20 years. Her interest in involving patients and the public in making decisions about healthcare and services has evolved during various research and development projects. The information and tips given in the book have come from personal experience of many of the quantitative and qualitative methods described. She has run focus groups and other types of small group discussions, undertaken many questionnaire surveys delivered by post, telephone, in newspapers or as face-to-face interviews and tried out consensus methods such as the Delphi technique. Ruth wrote the Primary Healthcare Strategy for North Staffordshire for which she consulted the local trusts, voluntary organisations, ordinary citizens, general practitioners and practice staff, other independent contractors such as pharmacists, dentists and optometrists, neighbourhood groups and the Community Health Council to derive support and consensus as far as was possible within the year's time frame.

Other influences in the thinking behind the contents and direction of the book have been gained from Ruth's time as Chair of Staffordshire Medical Audit Advisory Group, membership of the Royal College of General Practitioners' Council and the NHS PCG Alliance Executive and working with Jane Routledge, Christine Adams and Andrea Green who have developed partnerships with patients, the public and the voluntary sector on behalf of North Staffordshire Health Authority.

To Barbara Brown, my secretary and personal assistant
for many years, who would like to be involved in making
decisions about her workload in the ways described
in this book!

CHAPTER 1

Achieving a meaningful dialogue with patients and the general public

You have to be sincere about wanting to involve patients and the public in making decisions about their own care or about local health services for any such exercise to be successful. You cannot expect ordinary people to put forward their views or take part in any discussion if they think that decisions have already been made and the consultation is just a public relations sham. People were talking about making consumer involvement in the NHS a reality in the early 1990s[1] but nearly a decade later, little has changed. An evaluation of GP commissioning pilots has shown that few of the commissioning groups involved patients or the public in planning services or appeared to know how to go about doing so.[2] Community Health Councils, 'patients' and the 'public' had little influence on the decision-making power of the commissioning pilots.[2]

Even if those working in the NHS want to involve patients and the public more, the exercise may still not be meaningful if people lack the skills to do it properly. Trust executives and some of those working in health authorities have had some experience of facing public meetings or holding other consultations but most people working in the NHS have no real experience of involving patients or the public in healthcare, over and above their day-to-day interaction with patients.[3]

Involvement may occur at three levels:

(1) for patients and their own care
(2) for patients and the public about the range and quality of health services
(3) in planning and organising service developments.

There is a mounting body of evidence to support the advantages of greater user and public involvement in the NHS.[4-6] The National Consumer Council cites examples of partnership working between the NHS and users of local health services that have resulted in more efficient use of local community resources, more effective health services and more accountability for public funds.[4] Community development work in Newcastle-upon-Tyne has demonstrated how primary care practitioners come to regard the community as a 'key asset in creating solutions' and become responsive to the community's view.[5] The NHS Executive regards user and public participation as an important priority for all primary care groups (PCGs) for the reasons given in the box below.

> **The NHS Executive[6] believes that users of the NHS should have a greater voice and influence because:**
>
> ▶ services are more likely to be appropriate and effective if based on needs identified together with users
> ▶ users are seeking more openness and accountability
> ▶ patients want more information about their health condition, treatment and care
> ▶ involving patients in their own care may improve healthcare outcomes and increase patient satisfaction
> ▶ patients need access to reliable and relevant information to be able to assess clinical effectiveness themselves.

Successive NHS documents have emphasised a vision of a changed culture and practice where user involvement and public engagement are integral to all NHS activities and accountability to the public is more explicit.[7-9] The NHS is becoming more customer focused, where the 'customer' is taken as meaning a patient or user, a carer of a patient, a group of patients or people with similar characteristics or the general public. Involving people in planning services and making decisions about local healthcare does increase their ownership of the NHS and gives them more understanding of how the NHS operates and the problems it faces. Closeness to the customer is reckoned to be a key characteristic of an effective organisation.

The NHS Executive vision

'The needs of the patient not the needs of the institutions will be at the heart of the new NHS'[7]

'... making sure that the NHS responds more quickly to patients' needs'[8]

'The Government expects Health Authorities to play a strong role in communicating with local people and ensuring public involvement in decision making about the local health service'[7]

'... ensure that Primary Care Groups have effective arrangements for public involvement'[7]

'... rebuild public confidence in the NHS as a public service, accountable to patients, open to the public and shaped by their views'[7]

'... ensure that consumer involvement in the NHS R and D programme improves the way research is prioritised, commissioned and disseminated'[9]

'... patients and carers need to be involved ... in their own care and in the planning, monitoring and development of health services'[8]

There have been some good examples of patient and public involvement where substantial changes have arisen as a result of health authorities consulting local people about the direction of future plans, contracts and services. But many other consultations have been of dubious quality and not been sustained. Some of the reasons for this are thought to be that:

▶ many public engagement initiatives are really public relations exercises in disguise
▶ methods of consultation may be dependent on practitioners' and commissioners' preferences and limited capabilities rather than being the best method(s) for the aim(s) of a particular consultation so that the results are not as meaningful as they might be
▶ there may be a lack of commitment from the consulting organisation or healthcare unit to act on the views obtained
▶ unwanted results may be disbelieved as being unrepresentative of the subject population and ignored
▶ decision making may be based on the historical background rather than a needs assessment or true consultation
▶ public consultation exercises are usually time consuming
▶ the enthusiasm of the response from the public and breadth and detail of information they volunteer sometimes catch the organiser of the consultation unawares and they become overwhelmed.

Other barriers to consultation in general include a lack of funds and a lack of clarity about how to get good public representation. Individuals' lack of confidence, time, training and skills are some of the barriers which deter ordinary citizens from joining in discussions about the health service on equal terms. People are more likely to become involved if they have spare time, for altruistic reasons, because of a personal interest or experience or because they feel strongly about an issue, either being angry about a situation or delighted about the service they have received.

Meaningful consultation is still in its infancy. Precisely which patients and members of the public should be involved in which way, when and to what extent is still the subject of much debate.[10] The evolution of an audit culture in the NHS in the 1990s did encourage a focus on monitoring the quality of care[11] provided, but most such work involved looking at quality from the professionals' perspective rather than that of the users or non-users. In the early 1990s patient satisfaction surveys became the vogue, often focusing on hospitality elements of healthcare services, and involving those who were able and motivated to answer self-completion questionnaires. Although the NHS workforce is unused to involving patients and the public in decision making, others in social services, voluntary organisations or local government are not and have been developing their expertise for years. Learning from their experience should help to avoid wasting time organising meaningless consultations.

If an exercise is to be meaningful, it has to involve people who represent the section of the population that the consultation is about. It is not sufficient to just talk to people who are the pillars of the community who attend everything. You must find ways to seek out the opinions of ordinary people who haven't got time to go to meetings or the inclination to fill in survey forms. People in hard-to-reach groups such as the homeless or those who speak little or no English will be most unlikely to come forward and give their views unless you use an intermediary. Many consultations at present involve the most accessible people and simply mirror the power balance that already exists in society. Some of the most accessible are voluntary organisations or users' groups; their opinions are not necessarily representative either of the constituents or communities with whom they work. Although their views are important, a range of other opinions are needed if the consultation is to be more than a token activity. You will have to set up systems to actively seek out and involve people from minority groups or those with sensory impairments such as blind or deaf people. And if you do manage to reach individuals in minority groups, don't get to know them too well or use them too often, as your relationship with them will become too close and cosy and they will no longer be truly representative of their sort of people.

Real consultation involves a shift of power. Many of those in PCGs or general practices may not be ready for that. Until they are, any user or public involvement in decision making will be a token event. Moving to meaningful user or public involvement will not happen until there is a change in culture

▼
True representation?

where those in the NHS want to engage with people and respond to their views. It is still common for doctors and nurses
to assume that they know what is in patients' best interests
without asking them and that their own views can be taken
as a proxy for those of their patients and the general public.
The public will be more likely to perceive a consultation as
being genuine if all stages are transparent: the purpose is clear,
everyone participating is well informed, all information about
the issues is brought out and there are no hidden agendas. One
way to ensure that everyone can participate is to minimise the
use of jargon and speak and write any public documents in
plain English, whether this is about an individual patient's care
or management or strategy documents that relate to the local
community. If people feel that their opinions matter and their

views are valued and incorporated in the decisions that are made they will be more likely to co-operate again in the future.

Consultation takes a considerable time, because of the need to use several approaches to find and involve people who are representative of the section of the population that the consultation is all about and gain their trust. The majority of the costs of a consultation are due to the amount of *time* people spend planning the exercise, seeking people out, carrying out the survey or organising interviews, group discussions or public meetings. As well as these direct costs, there are the opportunity costs of the other work they might have been doing. The amount of money or time spent is not necessarily directly proportional to how meaningful the consultation is. Much money can be spent on distributing glossy pamphlets or holding high-profile events like citizens' juries. There may be simpler ways of gaining information, such as asking different groups of people already meeting in clubs or at clinics to comment on the services provided. Ordinary people often have good ideas about saving money and time, having witnessed inefficiencies whilst receiving healthcare. You may not need to invent new, potentially costly methods of gaining patients' or the public's views but instead extend some of the ways that already exist, such as by expanding the Community Health Council's role or sharing the systems that local authorities have set up. Although extensive consultation is costly it might be more expensive in the long run not to consult and to continue to waste resources on inappropriate NHS services.

It would not do for staff's views to be overlooked in the rush to consult patients and the public. Staff should also be involved in a meaningful way in any decision making. They will be as much affected by any changes or improvement programmes as the patients or the public will be. NHS leaders and managers have often neglected to consult staff in the past and consequently unrealistic decisions have been taken that might have been avoided if staff had been properly involved throughout and their opinions taken into account.

Establishing a more positive culture of user involvement and public engagement will require PCGs and trusts to win the hearts and minds of NHS staff to gain their commitment to really trying to involve patients and the public. That means taking their views into account and not just listening to them. And equally, PCGs and trusts should understand what motivates lay people (citizens, users and non-users) to become involved in the planning, provision and decision-making processes of primary healthcare and how they can be helped to contribute. This area of work will overlap with the responsibilities of those leading the PCG or trust on clinical governance and education and training matters. If services are to be shaped to patients' and the local communities' views, PCGs, trusts and health authorities[12] will have to develop methodologically sound ways of obtaining such views and encouraging local people and health professionals to participate.

References

1 Joule N (1993) Involving users of health care services: moving beyond lip service (editorial). *Quality in Health Care.* **2**: 211–12.

2 Regen E, Smith J, Shapiro J (1999) *First Off the Starting Block: Lessons from GP Commissioning Pilots for PCGs.* Health Services Management Centre, University of Birmingham, Birmingham.

3 Macleod N, Moloney R, Chambers R (1999) *The Education and Training Needs of Primary Care Groups: Supporting Staff to Meet the Needs.* Staffordshire University, Stafford.

4 National Consumer Council (1995) *In Partnership with Patients.* National Consumer Council, London.

5 Crowley P (1998) *Involving the community in primary care groups.* Abstract of presentation given at NHS Alliance National Conference, Blackpool. Contact address: West End Health Resource Centre, Adelaide Terrace, Newcastle on Tyne NE4 8BE.

6 NHS Executive (1997) *Priorities and Planning Guidelines for the NHS: Medium Term Priorities.* HMSO, London.

7 NHS Executive (1997) *The New NHS: Modern, Dependable.* Department of Health, London.

8 NHS Executive (1996) *Patient Partnership: Building a Collaborative Strategy*. Department of Health, Leeds.

9 NHS Executive (1998) *Research: What's in it for Consumers?* Department of Health, London.

10 Renn O, Webler T, Wiedemann P (1995) *Fairness and Competence in Citizen Participation*. Kluwer Academic, London.

11 Kelson M (1998) *Promoting Patient Involvement in Clinical Audit*. College of Health, London.

12 Routledge J, Adams C (1999) *Public Partnership Framework*. North Staffordshire Health Authority, Stoke-on-Trent.

CHAPTER 2

Using questionnaire and interview surveys to gather information and views from patients and the general public

You should be sure of your purpose before involving patients and the public in planning and delivering care, know how to choose the right method and how to use the information gained to best effect. Different techniques may give dissimilar results if the methods used are biased. Biases may arise if the sampling of the population is unscientific and the people involved are not representative of the population as a whole, if the questions used are ambiguous or if those participating do not give honest answers. If the consultation is about complex issues like rationing or prioritising healthcare, the participants are likely to need to be informed about the topic first and have opportunities to discuss, debate and reflect on the issues.[1]

This chapter will describe a range of different types of patient or public exercises and some of the advantages and disadvantages of each method. Some methods are more time consuming and costly than others but the outcomes might be more representative of what the general population think. To some extent, there is a trade-off between a method of convenience, which is usually cheaper in terms of resources and maybe more likely to produce biased views, and one where more complex and time-consuming methods are designed to elicit representative opinions from a cross-section of the relevant population. The details given in the boxes of examples not only illustrate the different methods but also provide additional information about how they work in practice. So you should read through the accounts of how the methods have been employed to get a better understanding of how you can apply the variety of methods in the real world.

These methods are not either/or. You will see that they all have different advantages and drawbacks and using one on its own is unlikely to give a full picture of views about the topic in question. The solution is to use more than one method to gauge patient or public opinion and validate your findings.

Questionnaire surveys

Good practice with questionnaires in general

Questionnaires are often used by first-time researchers as the tool of choice for finding out the answer to their research questions. They may mistakenly believe that undertaking a questionnaire survey is one of the simplest and easiest methods. Unfortunately for them, using a questionnaire is full of pitfalls and it is one of the most difficult techniques for gaining a true or valid answer to the question posed.

The questions

A valid questionnaire will have questions that:

▶ are relevant and appropriate to the purpose of the enquiry
▶ are unambiguous
▶ contain one idea or enquiry at a time
▶ have an easily answered format with simple choices of response

- flow in a logical order
- don't make assumptions
- use appropriate language likely to be understood by all respondents
- are not biased or leading
- are not offensive.

You should avoid leading questions that imply that you are expecting a particular answer. Otherwise respondents will tend to give the answer implied as being the 'right' one because they want to please the researcher or because they feel that their own view might be considered to be 'wrong' by others.

Use simple English easily understandable to a typical person in the population you are targeting with the survey. If any words are ambiguous or vaguely descriptive you should either omit them from your question or justify what you mean by them. If any of these kinds of word do slip through, they should be identified by the people in the pilot phase of the study. Don't use jargon. Avoid long and complicated questions.

Only ask questions that people can answer. You do not want people to have to go away to hunt out the answers as they are unlikely to return to complete the questionnaire and your response rate will be low. Similarly, avoid hypothetical questions as far as you can; it is well known that people do not necessarily behave how they say they will in advance of a situation occurring. If respondents have to guess the answers, your responses will be relatively meaningless, so only ask questions to which you can expect accurate answers. If respondents will not be able to answer the questions easily and accurately, choose a different study method.

Be careful not to ask two questions at the same time. This is a very common mistake. You will not know to which part of the double question the answer applies when you are analysing the answers. That's if the subject does reply, as people will be more likely to throw a badly constructed questionnaire away without completing it.

The answers

It is better to avoid using 'banded' answers in your questionnaire and ask for specific information instead. If your choice of banding is poor you will lose a lot of information if you find that most of your respondents are in one category; for instance, if you were to ask respondents' age as age bands instead of exact years, you might find that 95% were in the age group 30 to 50 years and you would not be able to make any conclusions about the influence of age on the responses they gave. You can always band answers yourself in the analysis stage. But you might purposely choose banded alternative answers for sensitive information such as personal income.

The types of answer will depend to some extent upon whether the questions posed are closed or open ones. The differences and relative advantages between open and closed questions are shown in the box. Closed questions give you a limited choice of options for response; for example, the range of answers to: 'How many times did you ring the surgery before you got through to make this appointment?' might be: once, twice, three or more times. An open question on the same topic might ask: 'Have you experienced any difficulties in phoning into the surgery to make an appointment?' and respondents might give more information about the time of day when there was most difficulty as well as the number of times the phone was usually engaged or the reception they received once the phone was answered. This richness of information is good if you wanted that information but wasteful if your open question triggers unnecessary information that is outside the purpose of your enquiry.

If you ask questions to elicit people's opinions rather than factual information, you might ask for answers using the Likert Scale, a visual analogue scale or the alternative faces type of response as illustrated in the box. Or you might present the respondents with a list of statements from which they can choose the one nearest to their way of thinking.

For the results to be valid and accurate, the respondents must be representative of the target population. The response rate should be high and as near to 100% as possible.

Drawbacks and benefits of open and closed questions

Feature	Open	Closed
Information content	Potential to be more detailed	Limited
Ease of completion	Takes more time, more difficult	Easy
Difficulty of designing question	Easy	More difficult to phrase to eliminate ambiguity
Ease of coding response	Difficult, more chance of error, maybe misinterpretation	Easy
Likelihood of unexpected response	Probable	Unlikely

Examples of different types of response

Likert Scale
5 = strongly agree, 4 = agree, 3 = uncertain (or neither agree nor disagree), 2 = disagree, 1 = strongly disagree.

Visual analogue scale
Respondents are asked to mark a cross on a line which best describes how they feel:
Very satisfied...Not at all satisfied
1   2   3   4   5   6   7   8   9   10

A delighted / unhappy faces scale[2]

▼

Have you experienced any difficulties in phoning into the surgery to make an appointment?

Pilot phase

Trying out your draft questionnaire on people who will not be in your final survey should detect problems with your questions or method of distributing and collecting the questionnaires. You should never miss out this pilot phase because you are short of time. Even if you are using a validated questionnaire that is well tried and tested it is still worth piloting your method of distribution and collection.

The number of people you choose for your pilot will depend on the number in your study population and how straightforward your method is. If you have a complicated study design and need to encompass minority groups, then your survey method will need to include sufficient responses from each of the particular subgroups of the population and the numbers of people you recruit for your pilot will be far more than for a simple study of easily accessible subjects. If you read published studies in the journals you can see that pilots often involve 10–50 people depending on the circumstances.

Benefits of a postal questionnaire survey

- ► It is relatively cheap as it does not involve interviewers.
- ► One skilled person can design the project, whilst less skilled staff undertake the data collection.
- ► Repeatable.
- ► Can be distributed over a wide geographical area.
- ► A snapshot of views.
- ► Can obtain the views of many people, although the bigger the survey, the more costly it is.
- ► There is no observer bias, as there may be with interviews.

Drawbacks of a postal questionnaire survey

- ► Chasing up non-respondents by post or phone increases costs and effort.

▸ Obtaining results is relatively time consuming allowing for time taken to chase up non-respondents and carrying out analyses.

▸ Response rates tend to be lower than for interview surveys.

▸ People who are illiterate, have learning disabilities, are visually impaired, have poor concentration, suffer mental health problems, elderly people and those from ethnic minority groups whose first language is not English will be under-represented as they are unlikely to complete questionnaires.

▸ The researcher cannot be sure who has answered a postal questionnaire; it has to be assumed that the person to whom the questionnaire was addressed is the one who responds.

▸ It may be easier for respondents to give dishonest answers to a postal questionnaire than in a face-to-face situation.

▸ No opportunity for the respondent to clarify the question if they do not fully understand it.

▸ No opportunity for dialogue or participation in decision making.

▸ People may be asked to give their opinion about services they know nothing or little about (see boxed example of the NHS patients' survey).

▸ Complex data collection and interpretation require good organisation.

▸ No explanation as to why respondents think in a particular way.

The first national survey of NHS patients

This 20-page postal survey of the general public asked about their experiences of using the NHS and what they felt about the services provided. Recipients of the unsolicited questionnaire were asked to respond with their views even if they had not had any contact with the NHS recently. Questions asked respondents for their experiences of access to the GPs, nurses and practice services where they are registered, whether a GP of the same sex as the respondent was available at their practice, how good their relationships and communication with the GP were, out-of-hours care and hospital referrals.

A protocol for carrying out a patient survey using a self-completion questionnaire

► Decide the exact question being posed.

► Write down the purpose of the survey.

► See if the information you intend to collect already exists elsewhere and if so, obtain those data and abandon your intended study.

► Define your target population.

► Consider the extent of resources available to undertake the survey: your and others' time, expertise in designing, coding and analysing, funds for printing and postage, etc.

► Write out the timetabled protocol: the number to be sampled (ask a statistician or other expert for help with deciding the optimal number needed), how sampling will be carried out, description of pilot phase, the method of delivery of the questionnaire (e.g. postal survey, newspaper survey, interview), how completed questionnaires will be returned, how and when non-respondents will be chased up, the outcomes by which achievement of the purpose will be measured, methods of dissemination, likely action plan resulting.

► Obtain ethical approval if appropriate (*see* Chapter 4).

► Identify if an established and valid questionnaire already exists. If so, find out if you can use it or must obtain permission from the author to do so.

► If no appropriate questionnaire exists, design your own. Carry out preliminary work gathering people's views as to the content and purpose of the survey. Keep going with your fieldwork until you feel that you have heard all the issues and are familiar with the language and phrasing the target population generally use.

► Frame your questions using the usual terminology favoured by your target population, making sure you will have elicited enough information in the questionnaire to be able to make decisions about how to progress afterwards.

► Set out your questionnaire to win the 'hearts and minds' of the respondents to encourage a good response rate; it must be attractively laid out, seem relevant and acceptable, as though it will provide useful information and be easily answered.

▶ Try to keep a written questionnaire reasonably short, for example two sides of A4, but don't achieve this by cramming in far too many questions in a small font size.

▶ Include a covering letter to explain the purpose of the questionnaire, what will happen to the results and how confidentiality will be maintained.

▶ Add the name of the author and return address on the questionnaire in case it gets separated from the covering letter.

▶ Do not include any unnecessary or meaningless questions: for instance, 'marital status' is included in many questionnaires and the results discarded because respondents find the question ambiguous, e.g. 'single' might mean 'unattached and available', 'attached but not married', 'divorced and not in long-term relationship'.

▶ Prepare the coding sheet for alternative responses.

▶ Try out the questionnaire on people who will not be amongst your sampled population. Ask them to tell you if they perceive any problems with the wording or the method or if any other questions should have been included and do not ask them just to answer the draft questionnaire. Check that the coding frame works for the responses you receive for both the open and closed questions. Refine your questionnaire and method accordingly.

▶ Number your target population and allocate each with a code number. If you write the code number in the top right-hand corner of the questionnaire form, then respondents may be invited to snip it off if they prefer, to ensure that their identity will not be known to anyone at all.

▶ Start your survey. Make it easy for respondents to return the questionnaires, with stamped addressed envelopes, a free-post address, easily accessible collection boxes, etc.

▶ Remind non-respondents once or twice, depending on your resources, time frame and how important it is to have as good a response rate as possible.

▶ Code the responses in the completed questionnaires; arrange for two people to independently code the open questions and compare how closely their interpretations of the themes and options agree, reaching a consensus where necessary.

▶ Enter the coded responses into a statistical software package such as Epi Info, Minitab or SPSS. The responses should be entered twice and any discrepancies between the two sets of results corrected. If you do not have access to a software package you can tot up the responses by hand but it will be more time consuming and you won't be able to do any statistical tests.

▶ Analyse the results. Look at the tallies summarising the numbers of respondents giving alternative answers to each question. Decide if you want to test whether there are any statistical associations between two answers; only do this if you can justify ordering the test and don't just trawl through all your data looking for any significant differences or correlations.

▶ Present your report with results that are easily understood by non-experts – perhaps as tables with percentages, bar charts, a graph or a pie chart. Include an honest assessment of the biases of the method and the limitations of the interpretation that might be put on the results. Add conclusions and an executive summary or abstract at the beginning that picks out the key points.

▶ Disseminate and share your results, change practice and systems as appropriate, feedback the results and any changes that are planned and have occurred to the respondents and patients and the public in general.

The covering letter for a postal questionnaire survey should:

▶ contain a brief description of what the purpose of the enquiry is, why the recipient has been selected, who is involved, what the time period is

continued

continued

► mention whether the respondent's reply will be anonymous or whether you are using a code number and if so, who knows to whom the code number refers
► emphasise confidentiality, stating that no individual or practice will be identified in any report, if this is so
► give a date by which you hope to receive a reply
► state how the completed questionnaire is to be returned, e.g. by a stamped addressed envelope
► thank the respondent for their help.

A rough time schedule for undertaking a questionnaire survey is about a year to 18 months by the time that the preparation, questionnaire design, piloting of the questionnaire, data collection and analysis and the writing and dissemination of the report are taken into account.

Patient satisfaction surveys

You might wish to assess patients' satisfaction with your practice, the PCG's way of working or the services available in a locality or a district. Doing patient satisfaction surveys became quite a popular pastime for the NHS in the early 1990s when medical audit was being developed. Patients tended to be asked for their views on their surroundings and how the NHS systems were working: what did they think of the waiting room, were they satisfied with the arrangements for making appointments or getting repeat prescriptions? Questions were usually relatively superficial and did not delve into complex areas.[3] Because the nature of the enquiry was so general, satisfaction rates were often high. The purpose of these patient satisfaction surveys was often to be seen to be taking part in the then-new audit culture, rather than to try and pinpoint problems and rectify them.

The new push to involve patients and the public in planning and delivering healthcare might have the same effect – of encouraging health professionals to be seen to be engaging in politically correct exercises but which may be relatively meaningless. Unless the organisers have a clear purpose and intent to make changes as a result of the information and co-operation they obtain from the public and others with whom they work feel part of the exercise and are willing to make appropriate changes too, they will not use the right tools or select the right methods. Nor will issues be probed at a deep enough level to give information about causes and problems to recommend changes that will make a difference in practice.

If you decide to compose your own questionnaire for a patient satisfaction survey, you should follow all the good advice on the content and protocol described above.[4] But it will probably be simpler and more valid to use a tried and tested questionnaire instead. Two questionnaires that have been developed for obtaining patients' views are given as Appendices 2 and 3 and the authors will allow them to be freely used by those in the NHS. The use of some questionnaires is restricted by copyright and requires a fee for photocopying them and surveying study populations. Some questionnaires can be purchased from commercial outlets with manuals that give details of scoring and comparable results.[5]

Before you start, you will have to decide what level of satisfaction will be acceptable to you. The specific level will depend on the circumstances of your enquiry and how important it is that people should be satisfied. It may not be possible to please everyone; the satisfaction threshold in a situation where you are asking a cross-section of the population about the allocation of resources that affects them directly, so that there will be some winners and losers, will differ from that in a consultation with the same population about a service that benefits them all.[6] Some feel that an 85% patient satisfaction level should be the threshold below which the organiser should be concerned about the level of dissatisfaction, whilst others accept a 70% overall satisfaction threshold.

You should already have ideas of alternative approaches you might take as a result of a patient satisfaction survey, so that you can follow through with a plan of action. People will only co-operate in future surveys if they see changes resulting from previous ones and don't perceive the next survey as just another public relations exercise.

A community mental health trust acts after a patient satisfaction survey indicates a lack of privacy

The Stafford-based trust runs patient satisfaction surveys as a regular part of its work. The surveys are just one component of a range of activities that encourage users and the general public to be involved in the delivery of mental healthcare. They work to a minimum threshold of 70% overall patient satisfaction.

A recent survey of inpatients identified privacy as a problem for some patients. The ward beds were rearranged to provide more privacy and plastic hoods were fitted to telephones sited in the corridor to allow for private conversations. Poor communication between some patients and the nurses and doctors looking after them also emerged as a theme of dissatisfaction. The care plan system was reviewed and changed as a result.

Newspaper surveys

Another method of administering a survey to the general public is via a free local newspaper. This has the advantage of being quick to distribute to many in the population. But you will have little control over exactly what is printed or who receives the questionnaire; it might be people passing through your locality and the newspaper may not be delivered to all the households you thought were covered. Nevertheless, useful information can be obtained in this way, as is illustrated in the example given.

Benefits of a newspaper survey

▶ Cheap administration, so long as the newspaper editor makes no charge for inserting it.
▶ Gain publicity for the issue as well as undertaking the enquiry.
▶ Quick method – no chasing up of non-respondents.
▶ Strengthens contacts with local press, paving the way for future articles on the same health topic when results are available, or other stories.

Drawbacks of a newspaper survey

▶ Low response rate.
▶ No control over who responds – some people may reply more than once if they pick up several copies of the newspaper, especially if there is a free prize draw to tempt them.
▶ Respondents are unlikely to be a representative section of the population.
▶ Newspaper staff may misprint questions or omit whole or parts of questions to fit within their space constraints.
▶ Non-English speakers unable to answer questions, although this may be partly minimised by advertising an option in minority languages for people to ring in for translated copies.
▶ Similar difficulties for poor readers, elderly people, etc. as for the drawbacks of a postal questionnaire survey, described previously.

A newspaper survey to elicit the general population's views about what the authorities might do to improve health in the city of Stoke-on-Trent[7]

A questionnaire was composed to test out the population's views about what the city might do to improve the health of the local community, based on previous findings from various

continued

continued

community development projects in the district. The questionnaire was printed in a free newspaper delivered to 110 000 homes and businesses and left at public access points. Prizes were offered to the first six entries drawn out of a hat after the closing date. Five hundred and twelve completed questionnaires were returned. Analysis showed that the age groups and gender mix of respondents were reasonably similar to those of the local general population. Around a fifth of respondents described themselves as being of Asian, Bangladeshi or Pakistani origin, compared to 3% of the local population being of ethnic minority origins, according to standard statistics. Respondents were more likely to be non-smokers compared to the known figures for the adult population, indicating a tendency to be more health conscious than average.

The most frequently given views, by at least three-fifths of respondents, of how the city might tackle poor health in the community were: 'targeting misuse of drugs', 'reducing air pollution', 'promoting good diet or nutrition', 'providing an antismoking campaign' and 'targeting alcohol abuse'. The most frequently cited factors that at least two-fifths of respondents thought made them less healthy were: 'too much stress or worry', 'lack of exercise', 'poor diet', 'very low income', 'fear of violence or crime' and 'animals fouling in the street'. These results are informing the development plans of the partners who commissioned the survey – the health authority, local authority, chamber of commerce, the community trust, the university and voluntary organisations.

Some of the main drawbacks to the survey were: the low response rate (which meant that the respondents were not representative of the general population, although the age/gender mix was similar); the printed questionnaire in the newspaper had many mistakes and omissions; not knowing whether people who completed the questionnaire fulfilled the study criteria and were adults living or working in the city (some people who responded lived 100 miles away, having picked up the questionnaire at the local railway station; some

continued

continued

gave their age as being under 18 years); and a disproportionately high percentage of people responded in an ethnic minority language because the person who translated the questionnaire into other languages hand delivered questionnaires to them and urged recipients to respond.

Interviewing

Interviews may be administered in person or over the telephone. An unstructured interview is an informal conversation initiated by the interviewer in which the person being interviewed describes their experiences and views. A structured interview is one where the interviewer works through a standardised questionnaire asking the questions in the same order and in the same way to each subject. A semistructured interview is also based upon a questionnaire but has a freer format in that the questions are taken in the order that follows the flow of the conversation. The interviewer usually sums up at the end of the interview, to check that the interviewee has had an opportunity to express their views, and invites any additional comments.

A protocol for undertaking a study where the information is obtained by interview is similar to that given for a postal survey above in that the same good practice in question construction should apply. The interview schedule should be piloted and revised accordingly. The analysis should be thought through when phrasing the questions, to make sure that the coding of questions for later analysis is relatively easy. The aim of the interview and context of the survey should be fully explained to the interviewee. Written consent should be obtained if appropriate, depending on the purpose of the study, the sensitivity and intrusiveness of the questions and characteristics of the person being interviewed.

The questions making up the interview schedule should start with straightforward, easily answered ones that put the interviewee at ease. The skilled interviewer asks the questions in an unbiased, non-threatening way and encourages confidences. Good interviewing skills include listening attentively, probing as appropriate, reflecting back what was said, noting and responding to non-verbal cues, showing empathy and being flexible about the depth and range of the questions, depending on how the interview is progressing. Biases arise when the interviewee is too eager to please the interviewer or alternatively takes a dislike to him or her. The interview should ideally be held in a room which is quiet, private and on neutral territory but many interviews take place in less than ideal conditions such as in a public place, for instance a street. Many interviews are audiotaped and transcribed to allow at least one independent person to listen to the tapes later and make a separate report of the themes and detailed responses that can be compared with the main researcher's version to reduce the chances of bias and misinterpretation of the interview material.

An interview survey to determine the general public's views about NHS prescription checks intended to detect and deter fraud

Face-to-face interviews were undertaken with a representative sample of 2047 adults in England, Wales and Scotland in one week of 1998. The object of the survey was to assess the acceptability of a change in practice whereby people collecting prescriptions from the pharmacy or surgery where they were dispensed would be asked in future to provide evidence of being exempt from paying for prescriptions, if they were claiming this was so. Two-thirds of the general public were 'very much in favour' and a further fifth were 'slightly in favour' of the checks on entitlement to free prescriptions. Virtually everyone was in favour of the government's plans to tackle all types of fraud within the NHS, with less than 2%

continued

continued

being against. The survey included open questions that invited people to say in their own words why they were in favour of the checks. The results helped to decide the content and message of the public information campaign and if there had been resistance to the change of policy then more information would have been given to explain and justify the reasons for the checks.

The interviewer should be careful to label the cassettes of the interview with the interviewees' names, the date, time, etc. It is useful to add their own comments and insights in brackets to the transcript of the tape, whilst they can recall them vividly, and highlight important phrases in the text – these might be new or surprising information, summarising points or phrases that are characteristic of the speaker. The interviewer may refine the interview schedules in the light of earlier interviews to focus down on particular areas or extend the enquiry if unexpected material has cropped up.

Gaining the carer's perspective[6]

Two hundred and seven carers were interviewed using semi-structured questionnaires, about three months after the people for whom they had cared had died of cancer at home.

Three-quarters of carers had not been told of support available from local charities and half had not been given advice on financial help. A minority had had difficulty getting professional help. Domestic help was often needed earlier than it had been arranged. Overall, three-quarters of the carers considered that the professional support they had received was 'excellent'.

Benefits of interviewing

- ▶ Better response rate than postal survey.
- ▶ Explores issues in depth.
- ▶ Interviewee more likely to trust interviewer and confide in him/her than to divulge sensitive information in a paper exercise.
- ▶ Can record non-verbal cues as well as spoken answers.
- ▶ Flexible questioning allows the interviewer to follow up interesting leads, especially if an unstructured interview schedule is used.
- ▶ Questions can be clarified if they seem ambiguous or unclear and if the interviewee has a poor grasp of the language, poor concentration or limited intelligence.
- ▶ You can be sure that the person responding is the person you are interviewing in a face-to-face situation.
- ▶ The interviewee is more likely to give an answer to every item on the interview schedule than if he or she were completing a postal enquiry.

Drawbacks of interviewing

- ▶ The social and ethnic characteristics of the interviewer may affect the responses.
- ▶ The interviewer may bias the responses if the interviewee is aware of the interviewer's own views.
- ▶ Relatively expensive in skilled interviewer time, travelling time, planning and piloting the interview schedule, transcribing and analysing audio tapes (may take a secretary up to eight hours to transcribe a one-hour tape).
- ▶ Analysing data requires interpretation of themes and content and therefore two researchers are needed to work in parallel to compare and agree findings.
- ▶ Interviewees may give the responses that they think the interviewer wants to hear, rather than honest answers.
- ▶ If people are being surveyed whose first language is not English, it is cheaper for an interpreter to translate a written

questionnaire for a postal survey than for bilingual inter-
preters to attend interviews.

Telephone interviewing

This is a cheaper option than face-to-face interviewing, as
travelling time is saved. Unless the interview is short, the interviewer may have to phone first to make an appointment to
conduct the telephone interview at a more convenient time. It
may be better to send a covering letter explaining the purpose
of the exercise and what is involved, similar to the covering
letter accompanying postal questionnaires, described before.

Some researchers have found that telephone interviewing
produces 'socially more desirable' responses than is the case
with a postal questionnaire method about the same topic.

Just as for a postal survey, the interviewer cannot be 100%
sure who is answering the questions on the other end of the
phone. Only people with telephones can respond and this
restricts the socioeconomic mix of the population included in
your survey. The telephone is a good way of including people
living in different geographical areas or targeting specific groups
of the population.

You might use a computer-assisted telephone interview
(CATI) technique to help gather the data.[8] This is a computer
program set up with alternative pathways of responses where
the interviewer is prompted by computer-generated questions.
As the respondent gives an answer this triggers the next appropriate question in the sequence. If you do use CATI, the interview schedule will have to be well structured and the pathways
of responses will need to be fast and operator friendly. Using
CATI makes coding much easier as it is done automatically
and the data analysis is very quick, so that the time taken to
undertake a survey is minimised. It is a relatively cheap way of
completing a large number of interviews and appears to be an
acceptable method of collecting information from the public.
Market research companies often use this method.

▼

You cannot be 100% sure who you are interviewing on the phone.

References

1   Dolan P, Cookson R, Ferguson B (1999) Effect of discussion
    and deliberation on the public's views of priority setting in
    health care: focus group study. *BMJ*. **318**: 916–19.

2   Bamford C, Jacoby A (1992) Development of patient satisfac-
    tion questionnaires: I. methodological issues. *Quality in Health
    Care*. **1**: 153–7.

3   Avis M (1997) Incorporating patients' voices in the audit
    process. *Quality in Health Care*. **6**: 86–91.

4   Grogan S, Conner M, Willits D, Norman P (1995) Development of a questionnaire to measure patients' satisfaction with general practitioners' services. *Br J Gen Pract*. **45**: 525–9.

5   NFER-Nelson (1999) Clinical psychology assessments and training catalogue. NFER-Nelson, Windsor.

6   Jones RVH, Hansford J, Fiske J (1993) Death from cancer at home: the carers' perspective. *BMJ*. **306**: 249–51.

7   Chambers R, Jacobs B, Schrijver E (1999) *Stoke-on-Trent City Population Survey*. School of Health, Staffordshire University, Stafford.

8   Harris D, Grimshaw J, Lemon J *et al*. (1993) The use of a computer-assisted telephone interview technique in a general practice research study. *Fam Pract*. **10**(4): 454–8.

CHAPTER 3

Working in groups, gauging public opinion, gaining consensus

This chapter will describe how to use a variety of qualitative methods to gather information and views from patients, carers and the general public. The methods covered are:

► focus groups: discussion groups
► special interest patient groups: user groups, carer groups, patient participation groups, disease support groups
► general public opinion: opinion polls, citizens' juries, standing panels, public meetings, neighbourhood forums
► community development: local community development projects, healthy living centre activities
► consensus events or activities: Delphi surveys, nominal groups, consensus development conferences
► informal feedback from patients: inhouse systems such as suggestion boxes, complaints.

Focus groups[1,2,3]

Focus groups offer a controlled method of enquiry into specific topics. They typically last between one and two hours. Groups are usually made up of between seven and ten people, but their size can range from four to 12 members. You need a minimum number of people to contribute ideas and a maximum number for interaction and to give everyone an opportunity to be involved. A moderator leads the group through a series of pre-prepared questions and themes, keeping the discussion constructive and focused on the topic in hand. If there is an observer, he or she remains outside the discussion but is available to advise the moderator how the discussion is progressing through the planned agenda. The discussions are often audiotaped so that comments made by the participants can be referred to and cited in any report. The person convening the focus group, the moderator, and the observer should have prepared well for the meeting and have captured the major issues as themes of five or six questions to be posed to participants. The questions should be framed to trigger discussion about feelings and attitudes as much as knowledge or experience.

The focus group should be held in a comfortable private room. The venue should be fixed on neutral territory if there is any question of a conflict of interests in relation to the issues to be discussed. Minimise external noise or any other intrusion that might distract the participants and disrupt the discussion.

Focus groups are composed of people who are similar to each other or share a common characteristic, such as having the same health problem, e.g. asthma, or the same experiences, e.g. recently discharged from hospital, or being in the same socioeconomic group. The topic, themes for discussion and participants themselves should all be selected as being the most suitable to fulfil the purpose of the focus group. It is best if the participants are complete strangers. Otherwise, they may feel unable to be entirely honest about what they think in front of people they know or will be working with. If some or all know each other, the moderator will have to take account of this.

The group moderator should be skilled at establishing a non-threatening and supportive atmosphere for the participants. Everyone should feel that their contributions are valued. They should feel reassured by the moderator being non-judgemental and setting out the questions in a neutral tone.

Rewards for participating vary: perhaps refreshments afterwards or a gift voucher for a nominal amount or as much as £30 for attending,[4] with travelling expenses reimbursed.

   The purpose and goals of the focus group should be clearly set out. The aim is to identify issues that had not previously been thought of, gain new insights about the issues from the participants' perspectives, gauge the strength of feeling about different issues and spot emerging trends. Focus groups help the organiser to learn the vocabulary of users which they can use later in a report or when describing the services for the public, to seem more in tune with or have more appeal to a particular user group, for example young people. The group is not expected to reach consensus or agree a plan of action or make recommendations. The organiser should continue to convene more focus groups to consider the same questions until no new information emerges. This might be by using the same questions with similarly composed groups or with groups that have a different mix of participants from a variety of backgrounds. Many people run three or four focus groups before feeling that they are not gathering new information but the exact number depends on the variability within the discussions and numbers of contrasting views expressed. The views of focus groups are not necessarily representative of the wider community, much depending on who was recruited to participate in the groups and how they were selected.

Focus groups identify the patient's view of the management of breast cancer in Sandwell

Twenty women who had been treated for breast cancer were randomly selected from the hospital patient administration system and invited to two parallel focus groups. The purpose of the focus groups was to hear about the women's experiences of treatment for breast cancer at Sandwell Hospital, in order to use that information to improve the service for future patients. All the women had undergone treatment at least 18 months before and were all physically well as far as hospital records showed. Discussions were audiotaped and transcribed. A clinical psychologist acted as facilitator and a nurse as observer. Eight

continued

continued

aspects of treatment for breast cancer constituted the agenda for discussion, which was developed by three clinical staff (the facilitator, a surgeon and breast care nurse), the Chief Officer of the Community Health Council and two staff specialising in clinical effectiveness.

A main theme of discussion for both groups was the importance of good information being given to patients throughout the care process: breaking the bad news about the diagnosis being cancer, knowing about the range of sources of information, having opportunities for discussion about surgery and its implications prior to surgery, making information and counselling available for patients' families and before providing after-surgery treatment such as chemotherapy. The draft copy of the report was approved by the participating patients before the final report was distributed to staff. Findings were fed back to the clinicians for them to recommend changes to the service.

Benefits of a focus group

- ▶ Gains insights into perceptions and feelings and the framework of understanding of the issues in question.
- ▶ Explores participants' attitudes, language and priorities.
- ▶ Information is gained over a short time frame.
- ▶ Only needs one skilled person – the group moderator.
- ▶ Relatively low cost – resources required for planning and preparation time, venue and hospitality for several short group meetings, compiling report.
- ▶ Can be used at different stages of healthcare: before (needs assessment), during and after a service is conceived and established.
- ▶ Stimulates debate.
- ▶ May include people who cannot read or write.
- ▶ Particularly good at identifying cultural values.
- ▶ People can participate who would usually say they have 'nothing to contribute' as they are more confident about joining in discussion as one of a group than as an individual.

▶ Can elicit views about 'embarrassing' topics.
▶ Participants can express criticism where they might not do so with another survey method.
▶ Good as second-line method to back up the results from a quantitative survey or to look at one of the findings in depth.

Drawbacks of a focus group

▶ Narrow purpose – focusing on perceptions rather than recommendations or action plan means that further follow-up work is required.
▶ Not necessarily representative of a cross-section of opinion or the population.
▶ Participants are not necessarily 'informed' about the issues being discussed and they might change their views if they were given more information and the opportunity for deliberation.
▶ Marginalised groups are unlikely to participate.
▶ Difficult to use when subjects are geographically dispersed.
▶ Costs can be higher than expected when the transcription costs of the discussions are taken into account.

Involving patients through user, support, participation or voluntary groups

There are at least five types of patient or voluntary groups: support groups, campaigning groups, social and/or healthcare providers, advice or information-giving organisations and the Community Health Council which is a statutory organisation. Few areas log all their existing voluntary organisations or map the different kinds of services they provide. In North Staffordshire there are more than 450 voluntary groups and probably others which are not known to the authorities. Some are stand-alone local groups and others branches of national organisations. Consequently, there is a great deal of duplication by different groups. Many people who might benefit from their help are not aware that the services exist.

User or support groups might be able to:

▸ raise general and specific concerns about treatment
▸ point out where complaints systems and services are not user friendly
▸ ask for more information about drugs and their side effects
▸ meet with the authorities or managers to tell them what standards and services they want
▸ help to train NHS staff so that they understand users and their needs better.

They generally offer support to people suffering a particular disease condition, such as Parkinson's disease, or who have a general problem, such as mental ill health, although a users' forum for mental health may not encompass all conditions such as dementia or age groups such as young or elderly people. Carers may also be welcomed and supported at user groups.

> **Users involved in training health and social care professionals**
>
> Mental health service users from MIND have been involved in training social services staff at Uttoxeter. To avoid overworking keen service users, the use of video-recorded user input is being discussed.

Campaigning groups or pressure groups may be a mixture of people with personal or caring experience of the problem or disease or well-intentioned people from the community. Their activities include fundraising, promoting the cause and high-lighting their key concerns through public awareness raising using the media, the press and any other appropriate medium, via schools and better literature.

Social and healthcare provision by the voluntary sector is of a far greater quantity and quality than many of those working in the NHS are aware. Health professionals are often surprised to find that voluntary groups provide healthcare from paid and qualified staff. Health authorities and local authorities commission health and social care services from voluntary organisations.

Advice-giving help by voluntary organisations is underutilised by doctors and nurses because of their lack of awareness and understanding of the services provided by voluntary groups. One example where the distance between general practice and the voluntary sector has led to patients not being made aware of potential benefits is illustrated in the box below.

Primary care professionals do not make patients aware of the advice that is available from Citizens Advice Bureaux with the result that some patients miss out on potential benefits

When CAB advice and support sessions have been piloted in general practices, substantial unclaimed benefits have been raised for patients on low incomes who have had no previous contact with the CAB services.[5] Some work has shown that clients visiting CAB services sited in general practices are more likely to be older and have a disability or long-term illness than those visiting traditional high-street CAB services. The take-up of CAB sessions located in primary care settings in pilot projects appears to be dependent on primary care team members' attitudes to working with external organisations and their extent of awareness, confidence and knowledge of what constitutes an appropriate referral for CAB advice. A way forward lies in finding methods of increasing the understanding of primary care staff and those working in CABs and other voluntary organisations of each others' roles and capabilities in enhancing patients' health and well-being.

A *Community Health Council* is a statutory organisation with a paid chief officer and volunteer members of the Council. There are nearly 300 Community Health Councils (CHCs) in England and Wales. Members are appointed by the local councillors and regional NHS sources and as representatives of voluntary organisations. They have a right to be consulted by the health authority on any proposed changes in the NHS. A CHC's duties and advice include: guiding patients through the complaints procedures; telling patients how to find primary care services; visiting hospitals and other NHS premises; and representing patients and groups and their interests with respect to NHS changes.

Community Health Councils were involved by half of the 40 GP commissioning pilot projects, usually in an advisory capacity with regard to 'public involvement'.[6]

Patient participation groups may be a mix between user or support groups, campaigning and advice groups, providers of social care and fundraisers. Members of patient participation groups may be invited or self-selected. The objectives of different groups include: involving patients in planning services; co-ordinating volunteer programmes (for example, volunteer-run transport schemes for the elderly, visiting the practice or hospitals); developing health promotion and illness prevention; providing feedback on existing services; and fundraising.[7] Some general practices have used patient participation groups to inform purchasing decisions for fundholders or primary medical service (PMS) pilots.

Patient participation groups flourish in some trusts and general practices but relatively few practices have such groups: there were thought to be about 160 UK practices with patient participation groups in 1996.[8] They are most likely to be successful when the objectives of the group are clear and there is continuous support from the practice or trust. The boxed example below illustrates the 'clients' council', a form of patient participation group in one community trust.

A clients' council established at a community mental health trust in Stafford

The council was set up in 1997 to involve and empower users of the trust's services, by gathering users' views and prioritising their issues. It has a core of ten lay members who form the

continued

continued

steering group and meets bimonthly with equal numbers of representatives of the trust – nurses, ward managers and trust management – to try and solve individual and group concerns. All of the council's representatives are either service users, former service users or carers. Most of the service users are outpatients. The council's open meetings give other users opportunities to express concerns or ask questions about anything to do with mental health issues or the trust, without any member of staff being present. Meetings are held in community premises and rotated around the locality. The trust is encouraging the council to become increasingly autonomous by establishing an executive core within the steering group to meet and liaise with members of the trust's executive team several times a year.

The Royal College of General Practitioners endorses the philosophy of patient participation groups and user involvement in general through its Patients' Liaison Group – *see* box.

The Royal College of General Practitioners' Patients' Liaison Group

The Group exists at the College to:

► communicate areas of patient concern
► consider ways of achieving a consistent and equitable quality of care for all
► encourage the involvement of patients in their own care and in the development of the health service at all levels
► foster relations between patients and their medical advisers on the basis of openness, equity, honesty and individual integrity
► encourage College faculties to involve patients in all aspects of their activities. (*Terms of Reference*, 1999)

The membership of 12 has a majority of lay people. The Chairman of the Patients' Liaison Group has a seat on the College's

continued

continued

council as an observer, but no voting rights. Their main concerns are that patients are involved in planning and delivering NHS care at all levels, in training healthcare staff, setting standards in clinical governance, helping with staff selection and training and contributing to guidelines about best practice and quality. They want to see the NHS take the public on board in a meaningful way in a culture of openness and accountability. Then, patients can expect to receive information about morbidity rates, be regularly updated about their progress, share information about the costs of treatment and doctors should not feel threatened by patients asking questions about their care or risks of treatment.

Gaining the general public's opinion

Involving the local community in making decisions about local health services should mean that services are better targeted at what the population wants and needs and public support for the services provided is promoted.

2001 census targets health

The 2001 census sent to 32 million households will contain three general questions on health in order to target local needs and inform the allocation of resources. The questions will ask respondents how they consider their health has been during the last 12 months, whether they are an unpaid carer and whether they suffer from a long-term illness.

Public consultation

Health and local authorities do hold public meetings if a major change to local service provision is being planned, such as closing a local hospital. But some public meetings are really public relations exercises, where decisions that have already been made behind the scenes are paraded as still being up for discussion. The issues raised in public consultation are often not explicit enough and may centre on establishing people's preferences, dissociated from the hard choices that would have to be made if new services were to be set up in line with their stated preferences. Sometimes the disinvestments that will be needed are discussed but as they are theoretical, they seem to be remote or apply to another section of the population from those being consulted. There may still be a public outcry about losing established services, even though this is a logical stage in switching resources to support the public's priorities.

▼

Public consultation.

Shaping services for older people in North Staffordshire by an extensive consultation with the local community[9]

The consultation exercise has actively involved more than 1000 local people. The local acute trust and community trust, the health authority and two neighbouring social services departments were all lead partners in formulating the proposed development plan following widespread consultation through:

▶ a series of local 'stakeholder' conferences providing opportunities for service users, carers, voluntary agencies, private and statutory service providers and commissioners to participate in developing the proposals by a two-way exchange of views and ideas

▶ meetings with a wide range of groups of older people with special needs including: people with visual or hearing problems, Asian males and females, an Afro-Caribbean group, people with learning disabilities, people from a Polish community

▶ local professionals including: GPs, a League of Friends, local councillors, non-executive members of the health authority and trusts, staff groups

▶ a questionnaire survey inviting comments on the report of the stakeholder conferences preceded by several meetings of around 300 older people organised by Age Concern and statutory agencies (435 questionnaires returned out of 2000)

▶ public briefings: a stand in a local shopping centre; press release

▶ correspondence with local MPs.

Some changes are already being piloted whilst the consultation continues as the proposed development plan is circulated widely for comments and views over a further three-month period. Older people are being recruited as 'ambassadors' to discuss the plan with various groups and report their comments. A further series of meetings is planned to review and debate the proposed plan with all those who contributed during the first phase of the consultation. Additional efforts are

continued

continued

being made to consult individual older people and their carers who do not belong to groups, using a 'carers' bus' as a way of contacting very isolated people.

'What You Said' – the responses to the 'Our City – Our Health' city-wide consultation in Sheffield[10]

Around 5000 people responded to this consultation exercise: 1421 were individuals, 90 interagency groups or organisations, 11 professional groups and 92 community groups. The aim of the consultation was to find out what people thought were the main health issues and problems affecting their health and to look for ideas about what could be done to improve health in Sheffield. The consultation methods included using facilitators to talk to people, groups and agencies, holding discussion groups, producing audio and written materials to inform the debate, appending a questionnaire to discussion documents. The responses were mainly written but included phone calls, memos, audio and videotaped comments and suggestions. The largest single issue was concern about the environment, with many people making links between their health and the environment in which they lived. Poverty and discrimination were both frequently mentioned as having major effects on people's ability to enjoy good health and well-being.

On the whole, consultation exercises fail to reach most of the population. Some public opinion exercises are targeted at people or organisations who are already informed about the issues in question – see the illustration in the box below of the Human Fertilisation and Embryology Association's public consultation on how banning payments to egg and sperm donors should be implemented.

Responses to the national public consultation on the implementation of withdrawal of payments to egg and sperm donors

The consultation paper was sent out to fertility centres and special interest groups across the UK; patients, the general public, clinic employees, health professionals and campaigners were all invited to respond. The consultation document contained background information about the topic and a mix of open and closed questions. The purpose of the exercise was to consult on how the HFEA's policy to end payments to donors might be implemented. The responses received were not expected to necessarily dictate the HFEA's future actions; they welcomed the information but reserved their right to take a different course of action if the majority of public opinion was not in line with their established policy on the matter.

In the event, 176 completed questionnaires were returned, of which 154 were from individuals and 22 were corporate replies from organisations, groups or centres. Responses were mixed and ranged from whole-hearted support for the HFEA's policy to accusations that the policy to end payments was out of touch with the real world and the numbers of donors would be drastically reduced as a result. Strong feelings spilled over outside the consultation to be expressed in the national press, too. The question behind the consultation about how to implement the policy was widened by respondents into challenges to the actual policy itself and included many other related issues such as preserving the anonymity of donors, access to treatment, the ethics and practical considerations of egg sharing as a method of donation and the importing/exporting of sperm to and from the UK.

As a result of the consultation and the HFEA's further reflections on the issue, the policy was softened and payments to donors of egg and sperm gametes were retained until acceptable alternatives were identified and introduced.

One cynic recently said: 'Money spent on public consultation is worthwhile if the public are behind you because you can make the changes happen quicker. If the public are against you, that just delays things for a while whilst you find another way or try again a year or two later'.

Open meetings of health authorities, trusts and primary care groups

The public is entitled to attend health authority and trust board meetings and this entitlement has been extended to those of primary care groups, which are subcommittees of the health authorities. Few of the public usually attend, although there is often a representative from the local press present. The Community Health Council does represent the public and boards are encouraged to allow the Community Health Council representative to sit with the board and be present at a closed session, although they would not have voting rights.

The government is committed to opening up NHS board meetings to the public.[11] 'Public board meetings should not be orchestrated events with decisions taken behind the scenes in a closed session.'[11] NHS boards should publicise their meetings well in advance and arrange their meetings so that the public feel they are welcome to attend and copies of the agenda and meeting papers should be available. Closed sessions should be limited to those areas of board business where real harm to individuals might result, such as discussion about staff disciplinary matters.

Opinion polls

Ordinary opinion polls, such as those operated by market researchers in the street, do not give the public a chance to form a considered opinion. Results given off the cuff may be misleading, as some people would change their minds and beliefs if they were better informed, as the boxed example shows.[4]

Effect of discussion and deliberation on the views of focus group participants[4]

Sixty patients from two urban general practices in North Yorkshire each attended two focus group meetings, two weeks apart. The participants' views about setting priorities in healthcare were systematically different at the end of their second focus group meeting compared to the beginning of the first meeting, after they had been given opportunities to discuss the issues and had time for personal reflection. About half of the participants initially wanted to give a lower priority to smokers, heavy drinkers and illicit drug users receiving healthcare but by the end of the second meeting, about one-third of these no longer wanted to discriminate against such people.

Deliberative opinion polls demonstrate that many members of the public will change their minds about an issue when given information and a chance to deliberate with experts and others from different social backgrounds. They measure the informed opinion of typically 250–600 randomly selected members of the public on a particular issue. The participants that are recruited reflect the profile of the wider population to which the issue applies. They are well briefed before the event which usually lasts 2–4 days. Participants deliberate on the issues in small groups and frame further questions to ask experts and politicians in full plenary sessions. The participants do not attempt to reach a shared view. Actual opinions and changes in opinion are measured over the polling event.

Other ways to inform the public include using standing citizens' panels and convening citizens' juries.

Standing panels

Typically a 500–3000 sample of the local population comprises a standing panel. As the participants remain on the panel, their opinions can be tracked over time. A sample of the population is usually recruited as panel members by post, telephone or hand-delivered letter. A proportion of the panel will be regularly replaced. The panel may be consulted as a whole by questionnaire or in sections through focus groups or workshops. Bradford and Lewisham are two areas with several years' experience of standing panels. Primary care groups may be able to use a local standing panel set up by others, as with the one illustrated in the box below in Stoke-on-Trent. Some areas have established several 'health panels' with around 12 members of the general public on each, who meet several times a year with the health authority to discuss health topics. Somerset,[12] Croydon and Lambeth, Southwark and Lewisham health authorities have set up a series of health panels.

▼
Standing panels.

A standing panel is set up in Stoke-on-Trent

Four thousand citizens were selected at random from the electoral register and invited by questionnaire to take part in the consultation exercises and help guide the city council's future work. The final panel has 650 volunteers who provide a representative cross-section of age, geographical and social mix from all parts of the city.

The panel's first consultation exercise was to revise and review the city's corporate plan by identifying people's concerns, needs and aspirations. Seventy percent of the panel responded. The panel members were most concerned about: increasing community safety and encouraging crime prevention; facilitating and encouraging the economic development of the city; raising educational achievement and opportunities for all people of all ages in the city; developing and enhancing opportunities to meet the social and health needs of the people. In addition, the panel urged that local action be taken to target the misuse of drugs; this was added to the corporate plan, having not previously featured as a priority in the city council's plan.

Citizens' juries[13,14]

Citizens' juries have been developed in the USA and Germany to give those in authority information about ordinary citizens' opinions. A typical jury has 10–20 people. The group meets to give a considered view on a set task, framed as a question. Jurors discuss and debate the issue in the light of written and verbal evidence from witnesses and experts before producing a report. The jurors look at the often complex issues from the point of view of a group of citizens rather than as consumers, experts or members of a special interest group. An independent facilitator is on hand to help the process. Citizens' juries have been used by local authorities to inform decision making and more recently, they have been tried in a health context.

Reports from areas in the UK that have experimented with citizens' juries have found that it was important to take time to decide the question to be put to the jury and express it in words that were seen as meaningful and appropriate to lay people.[13] Typically, jurors are asked to choose between options drawn up by the health authority or to develop criteria to guide decisions on a particular issue. Each of these citizens' juries[13] had a steering group who shaped the question, prepared the information and evidence for the jurors, identified witnesses, involved the 'stakeholders' who were likely to be the ones to take any recommendations forward and a wide range of others with a broad platform of interests.[14] In each case a project worker took 5–6 months to set up, organise and run the citizens' jury. Jurors were not elected by the local population but were recruited by independent organisations such as market research companies. They were selected to reflect the profile of the local population with respect to age, gender, employment status, ethnicity and geographical spread. Some organisers realised retrospectively that it would have been better if jurors had not known one another prior to the jury being convened.

The organisers learnt that it was best if witnesses limited the giving of their evidence to 15 minutes followed by 30–45 minutes for questions from the jury. A brief written summary of the information they presented was helpful to the jurors. A typical jury lasted four and a half days and jurors were paid £200 plus expenses. Most limited the numbers of observers to 12 and placed them behind the jurors so that they were less distracting. The most important feature of the venues where the juries were held was that the jurors, observers and witnesses could remain separate at refreshment breaks. The jury report was typically written by the project officer employed by the jury sponsors who were members of the steering group and not the health authority. The jurors approved the reports before they were submitted to the commissioning body – the health authority or local authority. The reports were practical and included recommendations for future policy and practice.

The outcomes of the citizens' juries piloted in the UK have varied from instances where the jury's report has influenced

▼

Citizens' juries.

local decision making to examples where the jury's verdict coincided with other people's earlier recommendations which then took on a higher priority.[13] The commissioning body should make the jury's report public and either plan to follow the jurors' recommendations or justify why they do not do so.

The evaluation of citizens' juries found that '... the cost of running a jury ... was a lot more expensive in terms of both staff time and cash needed than the usual methods employed to involve the public ...'.[13] The costs were estimated to be between £16 000 plus staff time[13,14] and £30 000.[15]

Some of the citizens' juries tried in the UK have been one part of a greater public involvement exercise, whilst others were a one-off event.

A citizens' jury hears evidence about access to health information[16]

Eighteen local people in East London heard evidence about residents' access to health information, from medical educators, health information experts and GPs amongst others. The jury advocated setting up health information points in public places, where people could get advice about medical conditions, where to get appropriate care, benefits and housing. The jury also recommended that health professionals were kept up to date about new information sources and that the NHS complaints procedures be better co-ordinated.

A citizens' jury debates who should make decisions about rationing[17]

Portsea Island Primary Care Group in Hampshire commissioned a citizens' jury of 14 members to give an independent verdict about who should take responsibility for rationing medical treatment. The jury heard evidence from GPs, health authority officials and MPs over a two-day period. The jury recognised that GPs could face a conflict of interest between financial and clinical issues but concluded that GPs were best placed to make decisions about rationing so long as primary care groups consult widely and are open and accountable to the public.

Benefits of citizens' juries

- ▶ May influence local decision making.
- ▶ Demonstrate the commissioning authority's accountability to the public.
- ▶ Keep the commissioning authority and experts in touch with the 'real world'.

Drawbacks of citizens' juries

▶ Time consuming to set up and run.
▶ Expensive.
▶ Involve relatively few people.
▶ Commissioning authority may disregard the jury's verdict.

Neighbourhood forums

A neighbourhood forum is exactly what it sounds like – a forum where nominated representatives of the local community, health professionals, the health authority and the Community Health Council come together regularly to discuss their local environment, health and housing issues within a community.

Involving the public through neighbourhood forums

There are 19 neighbourhood forums in North Staffordshire, with GPs, district nurses, clergy, school teachers, users, carers and many other members of the local community and NHS amongst the membership. They meet quarterly and are facilitated by a member of the health authority who also acts as a two-way conduit between the health authority and each forum. Typical priority issues are: the cost and infrequency of local public transport; drug and alcohol misuse; lack of dental provision; the need for community health promotion schemes.

Able and willing members of different forums come together to provide 'readers' panels' consisting of 10–25 people. On one occasion they reviewed and commented on a draft strategic document from the health authority, which they had read prior to the meeting. Their comments included advice about the user friendliness and readability of the document as well as the relevance and appropriateness of the contents.

Community development

Community development is targeted at people who tend to be excluded from society or who share a common characteristic. That might be that they live in the same locality or have a common feature in their lives, such as being a young single parent or living on the same housing estate. Community development aims to help people 'tackle for themselves the problems which they face and identify to be important and ... empower them to change things by developing their own skills, knowledge and experience and by working in partnership with other groups and with statutory agencies'.[18] It involves interaction between communities and statutory and other agencies, using consultation and advocacy. Those undertaking community development use methods like focus groups and observation to inform the developmental work and to evaluate whether it has been effective.

Trained community development workers bring local people together to:

► 'identify and support existing community networks, thus improving health
► identify health needs, in particular those of marginalised groups and those suffering inequality
► work with other relevant agencies, including community groups, to tackle identified needs
► encourage dialogue with commissioners to develop more accessible and appropriate services'.[19]

In particular, community workers may gather evidence about successful models used elsewhere and get interested parties to work together with the local community to see how such models might be adopted and funded locally.

All these activities are at the heart of primary care groups' responsibilities. Few of the previous primary care commissioning groups took on community development[6] or public involvement and so PCGs will benefit from working with established community development workers now to make best use of their

Evolving a healthy living centre from community development work[20]

Health and social needs of the deprived community of Chell have been undertaken through several community projects over two years that have assessed the population's 'needs' from an NHS perspective and the community's 'wants' by listening to local people as groups and as individuals. As a result, a healthy living centre is being created and will offer a gymnasium, a drop-in café, youth facilities, some community education sessions and multipurpose rooms for various community activities, community health services and medical services provided by a local general practitioner with a nurse partner.

The business case for the healthy living centre recognises that 'the local community needs to have a say as to how the centre develops in future'. The overall justification for the centre is: 'to promote collaborative work with the local community, to improve access to information and advice which can help local people take more control of their own situations and to encourage activities which empower and raise the aspirations of the local community'. The centre will involve the local community in its management structure and 'take full account of its views'.

skills. Champions of community development feel that the techniques could help PCGs 'develop decision-making processes that truly involve users'.[19]

Community participation in primary care groups and the health action zone in Tyne and Wear[21]

GPs and others in Newcastle and North Tyneside have been working with community involvement initiatives since 1994. The Newcastle Health Partnership has a strategy for city-wide community participation that aims to help local communities

continued

continued

act on their own health agendas. Special efforts have been made to include black and ethnic minorities, gay and lesbian groups, older people, adolescents and people with a physical or sensory disability. The community development worker in the west end of Newcastle is accountable to the local community rather than the health authority.

Health priorities emerged from the 90 local groups involved in the initiative and were taken up by health services management. The community worker and two lay members of the health action group have places on the local PCG's board. An annual local health conference is attended by more than 200 local people and develops priorities for the year's proposed health commissioning. Their experience is that public involvement leads to a greater understanding of local health issues and new ways of tackling them. The two-way dialogue improves relationships and gives the public an insight into the pressures on health services.

Health parliaments

Potentially, a parliament might consist of up to 120 members from statutory and non-statutory organisations and members of the public. The aim is to provide a democratic decision-making process to discuss, debate and decide upon a way forward for local strategies and developments.

A youth parliament

One health action zone that plans to put public opinion at the heart of all its activities is setting up a 'youth parliament'.[22] They hope to use the parliament to test whether they are making a real difference to health on the ground. The organisers have chosen this approach in response to the frequent calls from young people consulted during other local community studies that they want to 'feel they have a voice and are listened to'.

Different varieties of methods have been tried for involving young people.

- Youth councils, such as in Devon, where 20 members aged between 14 and 25 years are elected by affiliated organisations which include schools and youth clubs. The council is supported and advised by several council departments and the local education department. The aim of a youth council is to participate in decision making. Members may meet regularly or come together as a one-off event.
- Young people's forums, such as in Manchester, where the members represent more than 20 youth groups. They advise staff from the health authority and city council on the delivery of services to young people.
- Young people's networks, such as in Cardiff where 1000 young people are involved and have advised the Welsh Office about the contents of the Patient's Charter for young people.

Rapid appraisal[23,24]

The research team gathers information from as many different sources as possible about the needs of a local population. This will include reviewing documents held by different agencies and directorates of the health authority, local authority, city council, chamber of commerce, voluntary groups, the education sector, the Community Health Council and other reports from various community development projects, local general practices and official statistics. The researcher interviews a small number of key informants, who represent local people, professionals, different organisations and agencies. Focus groups and postal surveys may also be employed. The local press may help by advertising the presence of the project, attracting information, publishing the results and inviting comments.

Benefits of rapid appraisal

▶ A multidisciplinary team of investigators reduces bias from the researching perspective.

▶ It is community orientated.

▶ The different sources of information give many dimensions to the problems and a more complete picture than if the exercise had fewer facets to it.

▶ Interviewing local people and professionals ensures that the results are current.

▶ The approach combines three perspectives: of individuals (the interviewing phase); population wide (the reports, interviewing); and community groups (interviewing, reports).

▶ The technique results in a plan of action for the prioritised problems and does not just stop at the information-gathering stage of other public involvement exercises.

▶ Those involved in carrying out and participating in the appraisal are likely to own the results and be committed to co-operating with the action plans.

▶ The technique encourages closer collaboration between health and social care organisations, housing, education and the public.

▶ Encourages local networking.

▶ Enables the local community to be involved in decision making.

Listening to local voices: adapting rapid appraisal to assess health and social needs in general practice in Edinburgh[23]

The technique of rapid appraisal was used to build a profile of a community living on a council estate of 670 homes. The three sources of information used were: existing documents about the neighbourhood; interviews with a range of informants; and direct observations. The interviews and focus groups

continued

continued

identified six priorities for change, many of which were not directly health related:

- arrange for a bus to come into the estate
- create multiple small areas and dog-free zones
- run advice-giving and educational activities in the community room
- improve the running of local general practices
- ask the local pharmacist to be more helpful about collecting and delivering prescriptions
- provide residents with practical advice about dealing with their difficult physical environment.

The rapid appraisal initiative took 12 meetings of the development team and 45 interviews; in retrospect, the team thought that the first 25 interviews with ten residents and 15 local workers would have been sufficient. The investigating team comprised a general practitioner from one of the two general practices serving the estate, a health visitor, the local community education worker and two local social workers, backed by a part-time secretary. The team members allotted about four hours per week to gathering the information over the project time period of three months, conducting the interviews in pairs. Two focus groups discussed and prioritised the problems identified and explored potential interventions.

The local newspaper reported the study in detail and invited comments on the findings and proposals. The team concluded that 'an expanded primary care team can use rapid appraisal as a first step in identifying and meeting local health needs. It facilitates a multidisciplinary approach and complements quantitative methods of assessing need'.

Drawbacks of rapid appraisal

- Biases may occur if the majority of informants selected share similar views and people covering the full range of opinions are not included.

▶ Bias from interviewers/researchers occurs if they are unskilled or their own views, ethnicity and gender influence the interviewees unduly (see 'Drawbacks of interviewing', p. 30).

▶ The appraisal is carried out over a short time frame.

▶ Written documents and reports used as sources of information may be out of date (e.g. the national census).

▶ Reports of previous work may refer to communities by ward, whilst the appraisal may be of part-communities that cross wards.

▶ The project work is time consuming, especially if local health professionals are involved and undertake the appraisal alongside their usual professional duties.

▶ Much organisation is required to arrange the interviews, especially with those from hard-to-reach groups who may be more difficult to tie down or persuade to join in.

▶ There are opportunity costs for all those taking part in the information-giving and gathering sides of the exercise.

Inhouse feedback from patients

The practice or trust could encourage public and patients to use feedback boxes more than they are used at present by making them more obvious and publicising changes that have resulted from such feedback. As with other methods of public or patient involvement, the usefulness of the exercise depends on the extent to which the practice or trust enters into the spirit of the exercise and uses the information obtained. If every positive or adverse comment is scrupulously logged in a record book by whoever receives or overhears it, then a more complete picture is built up, rather than an occasional note of praise or complaint being received. A culture should be encouraged where it is accepted as being in everyone's interests that patients feel able to air problems and difficulties before they become significant complaints.

One of the components of clinical governance that should be highlighted as an important aspect not to be overlooked is for the NHS to 'celebrate' its success. Collecting positive suggestions and feedback is one way of achieving such a positive approach.

> **General practices involve patients in feedback exercises to design their Patient's Charter**
>
> One of the successes of Staffordshire Medical Audit Advisory Group's Patient Charter project was to encourage general practices to design their own charter with a set of 'rights' and 'responsibilities' that were realistic for that practice. Of the 55 practices replying to a follow-up questionnaire in 1997, 38 (69%) had involved patients in setting or commenting on the standards, in various ways.

According to a recent report, general practitioners are 13 times more likely to be sued than ten years ago.[25] The general public are said to be more conscious of their rights and more likely to sue. The informal complaints procedures in practices and trusts do defuse many complaints at an inhouse stage rather than involving the health authority, NHS ombudsman or General Medical Council. Any complaints procedure should be well publicised, speedy, open, impartial and focused on resolving grievances and improving services.

Consensus exercises

Nominal groups, consensus conferences and the Delphi technique are three different types of consensus exercises. Consensus methods may be used to help make decisions where there is an overload of information about a subject and some of it is contradictory, so that it is unclear what is the best way forward. The experts involved contribute wide-ranging information, some of which may not be published and would not be available except by talking to the experts. Their insights into the problem or issue being considered are as important as the knowledge they contribute.

Nominal group[26,27,28]

The nominal group is a structured group method used for generating ideas in answer to a specific question. The group meeting usually lasts about 1–2 hours and involves 5–9 people, although as many as 12 might participate. The structure tends to encourage everyone's participation and reduce any disproportionate input from the more dominant personalities in the group, so that the ideas and plans arising from group discussion are more democratically determined. The facilitator should be experienced in group work rather than be an expert on the topic under question. The purpose of the group meeting should be clear and the question or problem explicitly stated so that all participants are sure about the task they are addressing.

- ▶ *Stage 1*: Each participant silently generates ideas in writing for 5–10 minutes in response to the question posed, jotting down ideas as brief phrases.
- ▶ *Stage 2*: Each participant takes it in turns to read out one idea at a time in a 'round robin'. The participant should contribute their best ideas first. These are listed verbatim on a flipchart by the facilitator or another group member and as sheets are filled they are hung up on available furniture and walls with Blu-tack. Participants can link new contributions into others' earlier ideas.
- ▶ *Stage 3*: Each idea is clarified if necessary and discussed. Duplicate ideas are combined. The separate ideas are numbered.
- ▶ *Stage 4*: The participants vote for their most important priorities from the numbered ideas using a pre-agreed voting system. In one example, participants allocated five votes to the item that they felt was the most important, down to one vote for the item that was the fifth most important for them.[28]
- ▶ *Stage 5*: The group discuss their action plan and priorities in the light of the voting and reach a consensus about how they will address the original question.

Benefits of a nominal group

- ► The method generates many ideas.
- ► The technique is useful for identifying problems, exploring solutions and establishing priorities.
- ► It encourages everyone to contribute and avoids a few people dominating the group.
- ► Participants are equal members of the group.
- ► It is a way of involving the 'grassroots' in the decision-making process.
- ► Participants may be of mixed backgrounds, for example from different disciplines or a mix of NHS staff and patients.
- ► The written generation of ideas encourages the commitment of the participants in taking part in the planned action.
- ► Only one skilled facilitator is needed.
- ► The technique produces an answer with few resources.
- ► Decisions are taken at the close of the meeting.

Drawbacks of a nominal group

- ► People have to be able to read and write.
- ► Group members have to make themselves available at the same time for the hour required, which may be difficult in tight work schedules.
- ► The ideas may be ill informed or impractical.
- ► For the nominal group to have a positive outcome, those in authority have either to accept the group's solution or participate themselves to be part of the process.
- ► The nominal group would have to be combined with other techniques for a complex issue or one that significantly affected others outside the sphere of influence of the group.

Consensus development conference[27,29]

Consensus development conferences have been used in industry on such subjects as air pollution and plant technology.

Consensus is reached by a panel of 10–20 lay people who have been well briefed prior to the event. The panel sits at the conference where members develop further understanding of the scientific or technical issues, 'in dialogue' with experts on the subject. The conference is open to the public who may also put questions to the experts. The panel members retire to try and reach a consensus view and then agree the contents of an independent report. The co-ordinator of the consensus development conference should be a skilled group leader and a disinterested party as far as the topic of the conference goes.

The NHS has used consensus development conferences as a means by which health professionals can reach a verdict about best practice in particular health conditions. In two examples, 21 medical experts came together for one day to agree a consensus statement on the diagnosis and recognition of depression and 17 medical experts (most of whom were the same as on the first occasion) considered the management of depression in the same way, on a second occasion.[30] Specific questions were addressed by a presenter with a prepared paper followed by another speaker giving their viewpoint on the first presentation. An agreed consensus was then reached after extensive general discussion. The draft consensus statement was circulated to participants for further refinement and approval. The consensus was owned by the participants themselves, rather than the Royal College of Psychiatrists and Royal College of General Practitioners whom they represented. The consensus statements were published as guidelines for other health professionals. These consensus conferences were run in much the same way as those which considered air pollution and plant technology, except that a wider audience was not present and prior briefing meetings were not held as the participants were already experts in their fields.

Benefits of a consensus development conference

▶ A one-off event means an answer is available in a short space of time.

► Specific consensus statements can shape and catalyse action plans.

► Those in authority may be invited to officially review consensus statements as a way of involving those in power, such as managers, to take forward the agreed consensus view.

► The consensus conference publicly highlights the issue in question.

Drawbacks of a consensus development conference

► The validity of the consensus reached is dependent on the credibility of panel members.

► There is an assumption that the participants can produce sound decisions.

► The stricter the criteria set to indicate the minimum level of agreement at which consensus may be taken to have been reached, the harder it is to obtain consensus.

► Large-scale consensus studies need political and professional support if they are to be actioned.

► The validity and reliability of consensus statements have not been established.[29]

Delphi technique[27,31]

Relevant individuals are recruited, usually on the basis of their knowledge and willingness to contribute. They may be experts in the field or ordinary citizens depending on the purpose and topic of the exercise. Many Delphi studies used in the NHS in the past have involved experts or informed advocates, rather than a random sample of participants, but the technique can be applied in many different circumstances and using experts is not essential.[31] The Delphi technique is a postal exercise consisting of three or four rounds (usually) of a self-completed questionnaire, the results from each being summarised and fed back to the participants after each round so that they may confirm or amend their previous responses at the next round.

The Delphi process ends when the participants stick by their previous opinions and do not wish to make changes or too few participants continue to return completed questionnaires.

▶ *Stage 1*: Potential participants are asked whether they are willing to take part in the exercise. The amount of work, numbers of rounds of the survey and time commitment are explained. They should be asked to make a definite commitment to participating throughout all the rounds of the survey as the validity and reliability of the survey will hinge on retaining as many respondents as possible at every stage of the process.

▶ *Stage 2*: Participants contribute their opinions about the topic or issues that are being considered; these should be their own views, expressed freely, and then posted back to the organiser. The opinions of all the participants are summarised and grouped together. The questionnaire (version 1) for stage 2 is built up from these opinions into statements to be considered by the participants in the next round.

▶ *Stage 3*: Participants rank their agreement to each statement in the questionnaire (version 1). This may be a simple 'yes/no' type of response or a more sensitive answer that portrays the degree of agreement or certainty with which the participant is responding to the statement. The rankings are summarised and included in the next version of the questionnaire (version 2). The organiser should encourage as good a response rate as possible and this might be by allowing three weeks for the participants to respond with a further reminder to non-respondents, for every round. Freepost envelopes and clear instructions will make responding easier and more likely.

▶ *Stage 4*: The next questionnaire (version 2) is circulated and participants rank the refined statements in the light of the given summaries of the group's range of responses. At this stage they are being asked in essence to confirm or amend their answers to the previous questionnaire (version 1).

▶ *Stage 5*: Responses are again summarised and ranked. If consensus has been reached, the survey may cease, but it is more usual to repeat the process one more time (Stage 6) to see if any more respondents wish to amend their views.

▸ *Stage 7*: The final results are fed back to the participants.

Benefits of a Delphi survey

▸ Anonymity of participants.
▸ The democratic process is designed to produce a representative opinion.
▸ Avoids dominance of one or more participants – everyone has an equal say.
▸ Low cost as experts contribute through postal means and time spent is minimal.
▸ Enables experts from a widespread geographical area to contribute.
▸ Captures experts' insights and knowledge.
▸ Individual participants can see where their thinking lies with reference to the range of opinions of the group.
▸ Individuals can change their opinion when they have had time to reflect.
▸ Judgement can be expressed as a summary of alternative responses rather than as a consensus statement.
▸ Can be used to explore policy issues or facilitate decision making.
▸ Larger numbers of participants give progressively more reliable outputs.

Drawbacks of a Delphi survey

▸ Successive rounds occur over several months and participants' initial enthusiasm may wear off and they may not respond after two rounds.
▸ The importance of good questionnaire design is sometimes forgotten in the organisation of the series of communications with participants and speed of construction of the questionnaire to maintain the participants' interest.

▶ Anonymity may lead to a lack of accountability.

▶ It should not be used as the single method on which to base decisions, because it is an abstract method with participants reaching consensus away from the real world.

▶ Co-ordinating large groups of respondents can be time consuming and problematic (e.g. chasing up non-respondents, maintaining contact details).

▶ There is no opportunity for personal contact between participants for them to discuss or challenge views if they should wish to do so.

▶ Minority views or disagreements may be ignored in the summarising and reaching consensus processes and the holders of these views may become disenchanted by the survey if they feel that their views were discarded. They may consequently be more likely to drop out of successive rounds, so that there appears to be more convergence of opinion than is really the case.

▶ A paper exercise misses out the non-written communication of participants' views – tone of voice, body language, etc.

Informal feedback from patients

Simple measures often work as well if not better than more complex systems, and cost little. Even if you have not had much success in the past with suggestion boxes or books for patients, re-consider using them. Patients say that they would welcome the opportunity to contribute suggestions and comments if they thought that someone would pay attention to them, and they knew how to go about it. So make sure that you fulfil both these points when inviting patient feedback.

One of the automobile assistance companies distributes a comment slip to every client to whom they are called out to help. Travel companies do the same on their client's return flights. You might not want to offer every patient the opportunity to comment routinely, but a targeted enquiry occasionally may give you valuable insights into the aspects of services and care patients value most, or would like to see improved.

Some practices have systems for recording every informal comment from patients rather than confine collection of patient feedback to formal complaints or extreme remarks. Reviewing this information every so often at a practice or trust meeting can shape developments.

▼
Informal feedback.

References

1 Basch CE (1987) Focus group interview: an underutilized research technique for improving theory and practice in health education. *Health Educ Quart.* **14**(4): 411–48.

2 Krueger RA (1988) *Focus Groups: A Practical Guide for Applied Research.* Sage Publications, California.

3 Kitzinger J (1995) Introducing focus groups. *BMJ.* **311**: 299–302.

4 Dolan P, Cookson R, Ferguson B (1999) Effect of discussion and deliberation on the public's views of priority setting in health care: focus group study. *BMJ*. **318**: 916–19.

5 Paris JAG, Player D (1993) Citizens' advice in general practice. *BMJ*. **306**: 1518–20.

6 Regen E, Smith J, Shapiro J (1999) *First Off the Starting Block: Lessons from GP Commissioning Pilots for PCGs*. Health Services Management Centre, University of Birmingham, Birmingham.

7 National Consumer Council (1995) *In Partnership with Patients*. National Consumer Council, London.

8 Popay J, Williams G (eds) (1994) *Researching the People's Health*. Routledge, London.

9 North Staffordshire Health Authority (1999) *Better Services, Better Futures. Consultation Report: A Plan for Improving Health and Social Care Services for Older People in North Staffordshire*. North Staffordshire Health Authority, Stoke-on-Trent.

10 Healthy Sheffield Partnership (1997) *What You Said*. Healthy Sheffield Support Team, Town Hall Chambers, 1 Barker's Pool, Sheffield S1 1EN.

11 NHS Executive (1998) *Opening Up NHS Board Meetings to the Public*. Health Service Circular 1998/207. Department of Health, Wetherby.

12 Bowie C, Richardson A, Sykes W (1995) Consulting the public about health service priorities. *BMJ*. **311**: 1155–8.

13 McIver S (1998) *Healthy Debate? An Independent Evaluation of Citizens' Juries in Health Settings*. King's Fund, London.

14 Bryan J (1997) Citizens' juries vote to extend nurse roles. *BMJ*. **314**: 773.

15 Coote A (1999) Citizens' jury: a forum for health debate (editorial). *Update*. **18 March**: 485.

16 Safir J (1999) Citizens' jury in bid to educate public on health. *Doctor*. **1 April**: 8.

17 Woods C (1999) Citizens' jury commissioned by PCG: news in brief. *Health Service J*. **1 April**: 4.

18 Barr A, Hashagen S, Purcell R (1996) *Monitoring and Evaluation of Community Development*. The Scottish Development Centre,

Voluntary Activity Unit, Department of Health and Social Services, Northern Ireland.

19 Fisher B, Neve H, Heritage Z (1999) Community development, user involvement, and primary health care. *BMJ*. **318**: 749–50.

20 Green A (1999) *Partnership Commitment to Redevelopment of Fegg Hayes Family Centre*. North Staffordshire Health Authority, Stoke-on-Trent.

21 Crowley P, Freake D (1999) Reaping the rewards. PCG partners, the public. *Doctor*. **8 April**: 62–3.

22 North Staffordshire Health Authority (1999) *Releasing Our Potential. Health Action Zone Implementation Plan*. North Staffordshire Health Authority, Stoke-on-Trent.

23 Murray SA, Tapson J, Turnbull L *et al*. (1994) Listening to local voices: adapting rapid appraisal to assess health and social needs in general practice. *BMJ*. **308**: 698–700.

24 Murray SA (1999) Experiences with 'rapid appraisal' in primary care: involving the public in assessing health needs, orientating staff, and educating medical students. *BMJ*. **318**: 440–4.

25 Pallot P (1999) Trust me, I'm a lawyer and I think we should sue. *Times*. **27 March**: B11.

26 Delbecq AL, Van de Ven AH, Gustafson DH (1975) *Group Techniques for Programme Planning: A Guide to Nominal Group and Delphi Processes*. Scott Foresman, Glenview, Illinois.

27 Jones J, Hunter D (1995) Consensus methods for medical and health services research. *BMJ*. **311**: 376–80.

28 Gallagher M (1993) Generating ideas for audit: nominal group technique. *Managing Audit Gen Pract*. **Winter**: 20–21.

29 Fink A, Kosecoff J, Chassin M, Brook RH (1984) Consensus methods: characteristics and guidelines for use. *Am J Public Health*. **74**(9): 979–83.

30 Paykel ES, Priest RG (1992) Recognition and management of depression in general practice: consensus statement. *BMJ*. **305**: 1198-202.

31 Linstone HA, Turoff M (eds) (1975) *The Delphi Method*. Addison-Wesley, Reading, Massachusetts.

CHAPTER 4

Doing it right: boring but necessary

Before you go on to apply your choice of methods of involving patients or engaging the public, it is important to make sure that you know something about the good practice and skills required to achieve meaningful results.

You should choose a method to sample your intended population that will include as representative a sample of people as possible. This requires a similar scientific framework as is necessary for any area of health research. The protocol for the study should be determined before any data gathering is carried out and include specific aims, appropriate methods and declared outcomes against which you can later evaluate the exercise. Any study should have adequate numbers or there will be unacceptable biases in the results. The extent of scientific rigour required for undertaking different episodes of consumer involvement will depend on the aims of the exercises, the degree of uncertainty which can be tolerated in the final conclusions and the likely variations of opinion in different subgroups of the population being engaged. The resources available – time, money, skills, staff – will influence the methods employed.

This chapter will consider:

► how to sample a population
► how to gain as representative a sample of the population for your exercise as possible
► patients' informed consent
► access to records

▶ best practice in planning, executing and writing up a survey or consultation exercise.

The actual construction of a questionnaire and carrying out of a survey was considered in Chapter 2. This chapter is concerned with making sure that you use a sound scientific approach to designing a quantitative survey or qualitative study.

How to sample a population[1,2]

You don't have to ask the opinion of every patient registered with a general practice to obtain information about the availability of appointments to see the doctor or nurse. You can get that information by asking a sample of the practice population and looking at the appointments book. But to get an accurate answer, the sample you asked would have to represent the whole practice population. If you were to ask every patient attending a Monday morning surgery how easy it had been to make their appointments, you would be asking people who had been able to overcome any difficulties and succeed in getting appointments and who were able to attend the surgery during working hours. There might still be many people excluded from your enquiry who had not been able to get through on the phone or who had voiced their request in such a way that they had received a prescription or advice instead of an appointment or whose work prevented them from attending a morning surgery. And Monday morning surgeries might be of a different nature to those held on other weekdays when people had not had to store up their medical problems whilst the surgery was closed for two days.

So the sampling technique you use is very important as you are trying to select a sample that can be trusted to represent the whole population to which the question underlying your survey applies. The stages in sampling a population are as follows.

Identify the entire population connected with the purpose of the survey and the question you are asking

The term 'population' is the entire group of people or things about which you want information; in the example given above, it is every person registered at one particular practice. If the investigation were about the treatment of asthmatics, the 'population' might be all people in one practice with asthma or all people known to have asthma or all people attending an asthma disease management clinic, depending on what the purpose of the survey was and the question posed. If the investigation was about the accuracy or completeness of record keeping, the 'population' could be the medical records of all patients in a particular practice or of the patients suffering from the disease in question or the paper or electronic versions of the records.

Decide the important characteristics of your population that might influence your survey results

A 'variable' is a characteristic of a unit of the population. You should identify important variables that might influence your results so that you can make sure that those characteristics feature in your sample to the same extent that they occur in the whole population from which the sample is taken. For instance, you might consider that age, ethnicity and gender are important variables in patients that influence how they re-spond to questions about lifestyle, travel or access to services.

Think of ways to sample that are as little biased as possible

Try to think of ways in which everybody in your population has an equal chance of being selected for your sample. A 'convenience' sample usually results in biases as it consists of a section of the study population that is easiest to reach. This might be the next 100 people to walk by. There may be good reasons why people with particular characteristics walk by where you are standing: if it is pub closing time you might find that many people who drink a good deal of alcohol are included in your sample or if it is the middle of the morning in a town centre you might find a disproportionate number of people who are unemployed or retired, compared to the demographic make-up of the local general population.

Using a convenience sample

A patients' discussion group was convened by a medical audit advisory group (MAAG) to find out more about patients' experiences when they were referred from primary to secondary care, investigated, diagnosed and treated and discharged back to the community. One of the audit facilitators recruited a convenience sample of patients for the focus group by simply walking into four different outpatient departments and inviting one patient from each to attend the group. The four patients could bring a friend or relative for company. All four came and brought someone else too – a son, a wife, a husband and a friend. The focus group discussion went well. The chief executive and a hospital consultant from the trust and two local GPs were participants in the group too, which was facilitated by the MAAG team. Problems of communication were identified throughout their care pathways from when patients presented to the GP, to their visits to hospital outpatients, whilst inpatients in hospital and when they had been discharged home. Lessons were taken back to the GP practices and the trust and triggered a range of initiatives to improve communication to patients.

Volunteers are another source of likely bias. They often have a reason for contributing their opinion and might be delighted with a service or displeased with their treatment or more interested in a particular topic. Health-conscious people are known to be more likely to respond to health-related surveys. People who have strong negative views are more likely to take the trouble to respond to an opinion-poll type of survey than people whose views are 'middle of the road'.

Random samples are less likely to be biased; that is, those in the sample population are more likely to be representative of the whole population if a fair method has been used in selecting them. It is best to decide on the actual number to sample in discussion with an expert such as a statistician or someone with considerable experience of surveys. You could number your whole population and then select every *nth* person or thing, where 'n' is the whole population divided by the number you intend to sample. You could use random number tables to make your selection from a specialist book or an electronic package. Or you could pull numbers out of a 'hat' in the same way as tickets are drawn in a raffle, so long as every person or thing in your population has a number which is placed in that 'hat' and an equal chance of being selected. If you take a systematic sample by numbering every patient on a practice list, for example, and take every *nth* patient, you must be sure that the characteristics being studied are evenly distributed in the individuals of your population. You could not randomly select patients from a section of the alphabet because those with a disease or from minority cultures will be clustered with family names around certain letters of the alphabet.

Random sampling patients from a practice register

A GP practice in the West Midlands has set up a patient participation group by inviting 16 people selected by random sampling from the age-sex register of its practice population. Seven patients accepted the invitation to meet and have since established a group. This method avoided the usual biases of a patient group formed from volunteers who are unlikely to be representative of the practice population and more likely to be champions of pet causes or the more vocal members of the community.

If you want to be in control of the way in which important characteristics or variables are distributed between the sample and the rest of the population, you might use *stratified sampling*. Sort your entire population out first according to whether they do or do not have the characteristics you have identified as possibly or probably having an important influence on your results. If this was gender, you will have two sections of your population – male and female. If an important variable was thought to be geographical location, you might categorise your population as to whether people lived or worked in an urban, rural or mix of urban and rural settings, or by the deprivation index for their locality. Then randomly select the sample in the same way as already described within each stratification or section of your population, weighting the number you draw from each category according to the frequency of that characteristic in the whole population or the proportions you want to study.

Bias is minimised by random sampling and by using a larger sample in proportion to the size of the whole population. The minimum number that you should include in your sample is worked out from a *power* calculation. Before you calculate the numbers for your sample, you need to decide how certain you wish to be that the results are correct (for the *confidence* in a statistical test) and how close you want the results to be to the true situation. The probability of detecting a difference when one actually exists is known as the *power* of a statistical test. Statistical significance can be misleading as differences which are inconsequential from a clinical or practical point of view (for instance, change of a few percentage points over time in satisfaction with a service) may be classed as 'significant' from a statistical test. Confidence levels of 95% are the norm for scientific tests. *Confidence intervals* give an idea of the range of uncertainty about whether a value in the results of a study lies within 95% (for instance) of the sample values from the whole population. The confidence interval gives you some idea of how close the results might be if you studied a large number of samples from the same population and how much the results from the sample in your survey can be trusted or how likely it is that your sample is truly representative of the whole population.

Most people use a statistician if they want to calculate the number of items or people they should sample that is likely to give them a statistical result from which they can be 95% confident that they have obtained a true result. Defining the right number to sample not only ensures that you have included enough people or things in your survey and won't need to repeat the exercise if the results are inconclusive, but also that you do not sample too many people or things, wasting your effort and intruding on an excessive number of people unnecessarily. There are 'ready reckoner' tables or formulae that you can use to calculate your own sample sizes.[3,4] One example given for medical audit of a population of 500 patients with a particular disease, such as hypertension, suggests that sampling 217 patients would be needed for 95% confidence that the results of the audit would be the same as if all 500 patients known to have hypertension were studied; whereas 176 of 500 patients should be sampled for a 90% confidence level and 278 of a population of 1000 for a 95% confidence level.[3]

If your sample size is likely to be too small because you have insufficient numbers of patients with a particular condition or characteristic, you could collaborate with other practices.

Pilot your sampling method

Pilot your method on people or things which will not be part of your final study population. The pilot phase should check that the subjects find the questions used in the questionnaire appropriate and easy to answer and should also test the feasibility of your proposed method to see if the sampling system works and the resulting sample is likely to be representative of the population as a whole.

Acknowledge the likely biases of your sample method

Sometimes it is not practicable to sample your population without significant bias. People's characteristics are not always known, your contact details may be incorrect or there may be a flaw in your method of sampling of which you were unaware until the results came in. You could find, for instance, that different ethnic groups vary in their willingness or ability to respond and that you have underestimated the barriers of language, culture or access to minority groups so that their response rates are low.

▼
Consulting hard-to-reach groups is difficult and may be costly.

Ideas on sampling a minority group[5]

Sampling minority populations and minimising biases are difficult.

▸ You might use census data to identify and work in geographical areas such as subdistricts or cities with a high proportion of people in the ethnic minority groups under study. But the ethnic minority population living in high-density areas may not be typical of that subgroup of the population in general. You may have to sample from several cities if you want to survey various ethnic groups as many cities have a preponderance of one ethnic grouping rather than substantial numbers from a range of different cultures.
▸ You could use a name recognition computer program to identify surnames likely to indicate people from an Asian community but surnames of other minority groups may not be so specific to a particular subgroup of the population as to render this worthwhile.

Validity and reliability of a questionnaire[1,2]

Validity is the degree to which you are measuring what you are supposed to be measuring. Reliability is the degree to which you are consistently measuring what you want to measure.

You are more likely to gain valid and reliable results in a survey if you use a valid and reliable tool that has been developed and tested by others than one you have dreamt up yourself and not tested adequately. A lot of effort is wasted composing poorly designed questionnaires when a published 'off the peg' questionnaire would have provided a more valid instrument and obtained a more meaningful answer to the survey questions. The advantage of designing your own questionnaire is that you can collect exactly the information you want but if the information you collect is of doubtful validity and you would get a completely different answer if you repeated the survey on another occasion with the same questionnaire using different subjects, then the whole exercise is meaningless.

So before designing your own questionnaire, have a good search in the literature to see if you can find a questionnaire that has already been tried and tested. You can compare your results with the ones obtained in published studies to see if your population gives similar findings or if there have been changes over time. You cannot adulterate a published questionnaire and still expect it to be valid. Even relatively minor changes like removing items of choice from a list of options can destroy the proven validity of the original questionnaire. If you must add your own questions, do so at the end of an established questionnaire to have the least detrimental effect on its validity.

The appendices include two questionnaires (the General Practice Assessment Survey[6] [GPAS] and the Patient Enablement Instrument[6,7]) that are still being researched but which measure the quality of services that patients receive in general practice and patients' perceived ability to understand and cope with their illnesses and help themselves. The GPAS measures access and availability, technical care, interpersonal care (including listening, explaining, time, caring and patience), continuity of care, trust, contextual knowledge (how well the doctor knows the patient), practice nursing care, referral and co-ordination of care outside the practice. The Patient Enablement Instrument focuses on how patients are coping with life or their illnesses and their approach to health.

Ethical approval

GPs, nurses, therapists and other health professionals who are not connected to universities or working with academics do not always realise when they should seek ethical approval for research studies they conduct on their patients. If in doubt practitioners should consult their local research ethical committee when they are planning the study. The committee should be contactable through the health authority which covers the geographical area in which the potential study will be based. The remit of the ethics committee includes:

► NHS patients recruited by virtue of their past or present treatment by the NHS, including those treated under contracts with private sector providers
► access to the records of past or present NHS patients
► the use of, or potential access to, NHS premises or facilities
► the recently dead, in NHS premises.[8]

Obtaining and storing data

The Data Protection Act (1984)

This requires that all personal data held on computer should be 'secure from loss or unauthorised disclosure'. Personal data are any information about someone else and include information collected in research or interviews about named subjects. The data holding on computers in your workplace should all be registered with the Data Protection Registrar[9] but it is as well to check that the registration includes the types of details you propose to store. If you are working on the consultation or survey on your home computer, you should register in that capacity. The Registrar will need to know:

► your name and address
► a description of the data
► the purpose for which the data are being held
► sources from which data were/will be obtained
► people to whom data may be disclosed
► countries where data may be transferred
► the address where subjects can obtain access to the data about themselves.

Statistical software

If you enter your data straight into a software package that has been developed for processing data from surveys then at the touch of a few keys, the computer will tally your results, produce bar charts, statistical tests, pie charts or graphs of your findings. You will see that researchers commonly cite Epi Info,[1] Mini-Tab[10] and SPSS[11] software packages in published surveys. Epi Info software may be freely used; the others have to be bought at reasonable costs. You may be able to find out more about what particular statistical program might be available and appropriate for your study from your local university department, the local medical audit advisory group or the information department at your trust or health authority.

Entering data is best carried out twice over, especially if it is important that you do not make any mistakes keying in the data to your PC. Compare the tallies of both sets of results to see if there are any discrepancies between them and chase up and correct the reason for that. If the questionnaire has been set up for it, answers can be scanned straight into a computer. In that case scanning can read ticks and crosses placed in boxes, encircled numbers and hand-printed characters and digits.

Informed consent

People should feel free to decline to participate in the consultation or survey without feeling that this will prejudice the quality of the care or attention they receive from you in future.[12] Consent is only meaningful if someone receives a full explanation of the intervention proposed. In the case of a consultation or survey, you should explain why you are carrying out the initiative and whether participating in the initial exercise could lead to them being asked to co-operate with more indepth work.

The right to grant or withhold consent presupposes the mental capacity or ability to do so. A recent report highlighted the association between competency or capacity to be well informed and the degree of previous education and doubted whether there has been sufficient recognition of the inability of some individuals to provide informed consent who have educational, social and cultural reasons that limit their understanding of complex issues.[13] You should be aware of this and act accordingly.

Patients' ability to understand and consent to randomised controlled trials depends on their education[13]

Forty middle-aged and elderly carers of patients with Alzheimer's disease (average age 64 years old) were given information about research trial design in semistructured interviews, backed by written information sheets. Three-fifths of them could not explain why placebo, randomisation and double-blind procedures were used. There was a significant positive correlation between competence to understand information about participating in a randomised controlled trial and degree of previous education received.

Access to medical records

It is common to find that a researcher from outside a practice has unlimited access to patients' medical records once the GPs have pledged to co-operate in a project. This is not to suggest that such access is unduly abused but there is the potential for abuse and patients have the right to know who has access to their medical records. The sharing of information should normally only occur with that patient's consent. The Caldicott Committee report found that there was a general lack of awareness throughout the NHS of existing guidance on confidentiality and security about patients' medical details.[14]

The more that patients and the general public are involved in the delivery of healthcare, the better will be the discussion and understanding of what constitutes acceptable limits to access of patients' medical records for the purposes of professional development and the measurement of effectiveness of the services provided and performance of individual practitioners.

Confidentiality

You should tell those you invite to participate the extent to which their identity, contact details and the information they give you are confidential to you, your work team or your organisation. If you are running a focus group or other small group work, you should suggest a code of practice to the group and seek their agreement or invite the group to decide their own rules. These will include agreement about confidentiality, exactly what information may or may not be repeated outside the group or if information may be freely repeated so long as it is not attributed to named individuals.

The Caldicott Committee report has described principles of good practice to safeguard patients' confidentiality when information is being used for non-clinical purposes.

▶ Justify the purpose.
▶ Do not use patient-identifiable information unless it is absolutely necessary.
▶ Use the minimum necessary patient-identifiable information.
▶ Access to patient-identifiable information should be on a strict need-to-know basis.
▶ Everyone with access to patient-identifiable information should be aware of their responsibilities.[14]

Template to evaluate the extent to which best practice was employed in undertaking a consultation exercise or survey

1 Is there a comprehensive report of the consultation/survey?

Check whether:

▶ it is written
▶ all stages of the consultation/survey are described; is there a stated purpose, aim, method, results, discussion, conclusions, recommendations, forward action plan?

- the choice of method can be justified
- outcome measures were specified at the start of the consultation/survey
- the details of the method are sufficiently full and clear that it could be duplicated if another person followed the report
- the results are presented in an easily understandable format. Do they seem to be complete?
- there is a discussion of the existence and influence of biases on the results. Is the consultation/survey set into context of previous work or others' studies elsewhere?
- the recommendations follow logically from the results of the consultation/survey
- ethical approval was sought and obtained (if appropriate).

2 How biased was the consultation or survey method?

Look at the following.

- The extent to which the patients, citizens or groups sampled were representative of the target population. To what extent did the subjects included in the consultation/survey come from particular disease groups, locality or population rather than representing a cross-section of the population central to the question?
- The processes by which the citizens/subjects were involved; for example, were they sampled, elected, nominated? To what extent did everyone in the population have an equal or fair chance of being selected to take part in the consultation/ survey?
- The response rates. Did sufficient numbers of people respond to give a reasonable chance that a full range of views was given?
- The distribution of age groups, gender, social class, employment status, any other important socioeconomic characteristics between respondents and non-respondents. Were the respondents representative of the whole population being consulted or surveyed?

▶ Did the consultation or survey method favour representatives with particular skills or characteristics (for example,
   were those without glasses or with poor communication
   skills less able to contribute)?
▶ Did the leader of the consultation/survey recognise the
   existence of particular biases in the final report?
▶ Had the leader of the consultation/survey tried to minimise
   the biases?
▶ Was the extent of bias resulting from the consultation/survey
   method acceptable?

3 Was the method that was set up appropriate?

Check the extent to which this was so:

▶ for the issues consulted upon
▶ for gathering responses that satisfied the purpose
▶ to match the intended outcomes
▶ for contributing patient/public opinion and views at an early
   enough stage in the decision-making process
▶ to gather sufficient information to know how to proceed
   after the consultation.

4 Was the information gathered used effectively?

Check if:

▶ there were any changes made from feeding results into the
   planning or provision of the healthcare process
▶ the target population, professionals or the authorities were
   consulted about the results of the consultation/survey and
   proposed changes to planning or provision
▶ there were any conflicts of interests (e.g. competing priorities); were they recognised, were they considered and how
   were they resolved?
▶ the dialogue with users, carers and the public continued
   after the results were published

▶ the report and results were disseminated widely to all the relevant people and organisations by appropriate means.

5 Was the consultation worthwhile?

Think about:

▶ whether the information was already available from other sources
▶ the realism of the resource consequences of the consultation
▶ the appropriateness of the costs of the consultation process
▶ whether the consultation process was a one-off event or part of a systematic or dynamic process
▶ whether the source of the resources used was appropriate for the purpose and outcome of the consultation/survey
▶ whether the opportunity costs arising from allocating the resources to undertake the consultation/survey were justified by the purpose and outcomes of the exercise
▶ whether there were sufficient resources to carry out a well-constructed consultation/survey or if limited resources led to cutting of corners that devalued the consultation/survey to a significant degree
▶ the extent to which the results of the consultation/survey were generalisable to other groups of people, populations, settings or circumstances.

6 Could the method of the consultation/survey be improved or response rate increased on a future occasion?

Consider:

▶ what facilitated or inhibited involvement of subjects in the consultation/survey and professionals or managers in undertaking the survey or implementing the recommendations that arose from the exercise

▸ what the benefits and drawbacks of involvement of patients or the public were as regards the purpose of the consultation/survey

▸ who else might have been involved to improve the information gathering and increase ownership of results and acceptance of change.

References

1 Armstrong R, Grace J (1994) *Research Methods and Audit in General Practice*. Oxford University Press, Oxford.

2 Carter Y, Thomas C (eds) (1997) *Research Methods in Primary Care*. Radcliffe Medical Press, Oxford.

3 Derry J (1993) Sample size for audit. *Managing Audit Gen Pract*. **Summer**: 17–20.

4 du Florey V (1993) Sample size for beginners. *BMJ*. **306**: 1181–4.

5 Office of Population Censuses and Surveys (1995). *Briefing 2*. NHS Health Survey Advice Centre, OPCS, London.

6 Roland M, Holden J, Campbell S (1999) *Quality Assessment for General Practice: Supporting Clinical Governance in Primary Care Groups*. National Primary Care Research and Development Centre, University of Manchester.

7 Howie JGR, Heaney D, Maxwell M, Walker JJ (1998) A comparison of the Patient Enablement Instrument (PEI) against two established satisfaction scales as an outcome measure of primary care consultations. *Fam Pract*. **15**: 165–71.

8 North Staffordshire Health Authority (1999) *Terms of Reference: Local Research Ethics Committee*. North Staffordshire Health Authority, Stoke-on-Trent.

9 The Data Protection Registrar, Wycliffe House, Water Lane, Wilmslow, Cheshire SK9 5AF. Tel: 01625 545745.

10 CleCom, Research Park, 97 Vincent Drive, Birmingham B15 2SQ.

11 SPSS UK Ltd, SPSS House, London Street, Chertsey, KT16 8AP.

12 General Medical Council (1998) *Seeking Patients' Consent: The Ethical Considerations*. General Medical Council, London.

13 Pucci E, Belardinelli N, Signorino M (1999) Patients' understanding of randomised controlled trials depends on their education (letter). *BMJ*. **318**: 875.

14 Department of Health (1997) *Report on the Review of Patient-Identifiable Information (The Caldicott Committee Report)*. Department of Health, London.

Further reading

Bowling A (1994) *Measuring Health*. Open University Press, Milton Keynes.

Calder J (1998) *Survey Research Methods*. Medical Education Booklet No. 2. Association for the Study of Medical Education (ASME), The Lister Institute, 11 Hill Square, Edinburgh EH8 9DR.

Moore D (1997) *Statistics, Concepts and Controversies* (4e). Freeman, New York.

CHAPTER 5

Choosing the right method for the right reasons

By now, you should know why you are involving patients and the public in healthcare and you have been introduced to the wide range of methods that people have tried with varying degrees of success. The next stage is to be able to decide which methods are the most appropriate for any particular situation.

There are four stages of thinking and preparation before you even embark on the process of involving users or engaging the public at large.

1 Take stock: be sure why you should do it at all.
2 Map out the skills and strengths of your team to assess the baseline to build on.
3 Assess the extent to which user involvement and public engagement are welcomed as a meaningful exercise by your colleagues at work. How much practical and emotional support will there be from others?
4 Before you start: define the purpose; be realistic about the magnitude of the planned exercise; select an appropriate method or several methods depending on the target population and your resources; get the commitment of everyone who will be affected by the exercise; frame the method in accordance with your perspective; write the protocol.

Stage 1: Take stock – why do it at all?

Don't just do a survey or run a focus group because it seems a good idea or there is a requirement to do it or it will end up as a meaningless exercise at the expense of your time and need-lessly raise other people's expectations about the possibility of change. So reflect on the following.

► Why are you considering organising a user involvement or public engagement exercise – what is the purpose of the exercise?

► Whose idea is it really? How many people in your practice or PCG or trust are backing the purpose of the exercise and own the initiative?

► Does the exercise need doing anyway? Is someone else already doing something similar and if so, can you adopt their results or tag onto their activity? Does the information already exist elsewhere that would answer the purpose of your exercise?

► Why are you considering being involved ? Is it your job to be involved? Have you free time in which to do it or can you stop doing something else instead? Could you get someone else at your workplace to do it? Or could you get someone else from outside your workplace to do it; for example, might the local MAAG or clinical audit department at your trust undertake the task as part of their job or is it a responsibility that the Community Health Council could take on?

► Would the exercise or activity be one part of the organ-isation's strategy – the business plan or the development plan? Would the task fall within a topic identified as a work-based priority or a local, district or national priority?

Stage 2: Map out your skills and strengths for setting up a user involvement or public engagement exercise

► Map out the skills you have within your work team; think of what personnel might be involved and who has skills to plan the exercise, type up any survey forms, gather data, analyse data, write up the report, action the findings? Does anyone in your work team have experience of doing anything similar or relevant in the past? Is there a local university or academic department who might help with the thinking behind the planning or the execution of the exercise?

► Assess the enthusiasm for the exercise. Discuss the prospect at an informal staff meeting or in day-to-day contact or at a business meeting of the practice or PCG or trust to see who is likely to be co-operative.

► What funds do you have at your disposable? Is there any specific money available or protected staff time or has any exercise to be added as an extra to everyone's workload? Are there any patients or members of the general public who might volunteer to help without charge? When working out the costings, remember to include the opportunity costs – the work that staff will not be doing if they are participating in the exercise or carrying out a task for the project.

► How well organised is your practice, PCG or trust? Have you already collected information about access, availability of services, patients' usage or morbidity data that is accurate and valid? Could that information be a sound base for planning user involvement and public engagement?

► What structures do you already have in place for undertaking user involvement or public engagement exercises? Do you have patient or user groups? Do lay people participate in planning services, training of staff, monitoring quality or communicating information in a way that you could extend or will you be starting from scratch? Are you networking with voluntary organisations or the Community Health Council?

► Are there any good models in your workplace or in neighbouring units or practices of user involvement or public engagement that include joint working between managers, clinicians, support staff and lay people on any issues that you could duplicate or from which you could learn?

► What is the quality of your existing patient information and education materials? Has anyone recently checked whether they are up to date, relevant and appropriate? Does the material you've got cater for people with special social or cultural needs and cover all their requirements?

Stage 3: Do your colleagues value the patients' or public's views? Do they believe that user involvement and public engagement is a meaningful exercise?

► Is there a culture of wanting to establish or maintain meaningful user involvement or public engagement or do colleagues see your plans as a paper exercise?

► Will there be resistance from colleagues to the exercise? What will be the extent of their co-operation or active resistance to the initiative? Is it you on your own or a team or is the drive to engage in this work coming from the organisation?

► Are the advantages to be gained from public engagement or user involvement clear to you and your colleagues?

► Are you and your colleagues aware of the drawbacks of public engagement or user involvement in respect of your particular planned exercise(s)?

► What are your and other colleagues' expectations of the usefulness of any exercise? Do you/they have positive expectations and anticipate the exercise leading to useful improvements? Or do you/they expect negative outcomes such as increasing patient demands or the staff workload?

► Do you or other colleagues have preconceived views about the willingness or ability of your patient population or the general community to co-operate and participate in user involvement or public engagement exercises? Do you/they have preferences for the population groups with which you prefer to work? Will there be any prejudices to overcome or difficulties to surmount amongst the staff – social, cultural, educational, lifestyle, etc?

Stage 4: How to start – making it happen

► Agree the purpose of the exercise with all your colleagues at work who will be affected by the exercise – either in the planning, organising, gathering of data, affording the costs, using the findings, working with the users or the general public, publicising the exercise or outcomes, etc.

► Define the question or the purpose of your exercise. Is it about:
  – improving information or communication or establishing people's preferences?
  – making difficult decisions about funding or resources; rationing or prioritising services; changing the availability of services, personnel or premises?
  – clinical governance; monitoring or improving the quality of clinical care or services?
  – assessing and targeting needs; containing demand?

► Be realistic in your choice of method depending on whether:
  – you have identified resources: skills, practical support, people, time, money, experience, enthusiasm
  – your practice or organisation and colleagues are behind you
  – you are capitalising on momentum created by the strategy at work or it being a priority
  – you are building on successful previous initiatives.

► Select an appropriate method for the population concerned:
  – the whole practice population or local community (users and non-users of your healthcare services)
  – identifiable patient groups
  – individual patients, carers or families.

► Frame the method depending on whether the exercise is to be from the perspective of:
  – a health authority or district
  – a primary care group or trust
  – a practice, department or clinic
  – an individual practitioner or member of staff.

► Write down the protocol for the exercise to include:
  – the purpose
  – the target population
  – the chosen method: how to sample or recruit lay people and professionals, the details of all the stages of the method – where, when, how many, who will do what
  – how other colleagues will be involved: how they will participate or how you will keep them informed and motivated

- – any training needs or skill deficits: how these will be addressed
- – the timetable
- – expected outcomes
- – resources, anticipated budget including time, staff, costs
- – context of the exercise: whether it is a one-off event or part of a programme of involvement/engagement or a preliminary stage to further work
- – method of evaluation
- – anticipated changes: possible alternatives that are realistic, acceptable, appropriate
- – expected dissemination: how you will feedback the outcomes of the exercise to the target population, those who participated in the exercise, the community at large, your work team, the health authority, etc.

▶ Arrange educational programmes as necessary for (i) those working in primary and community healthcare and the voluntary sector and (ii) members of the public, users and carers to learn how to initiate or participate in lay consultation/involvement, to make the most of resources or opportunities and use the results of the consultation effectively.

Stage 5: Involving patients and the public appropriately

Use the lists of alternatives below to help you decide what method(s) you will use. There are many varied examples to illustrate the sort of objectives, topics or themes for the type of patient or general public populations with which you might work. The objectives, topics, populations and methods described are by no means comprehensive, they are just intended to give you examples of the kind of approaches you should consider. Your own circumstances will limit your choice of methods for all the reasons previously listed above. The characteristics of your local population and the quality of the current provision of services will shape your purpose and the subsidiary objectives of the patient or public information and involvement activities on which you embark; they may be completely different from any illustrated here.

Refer back to the previous chapters for descriptions of the different types of involvement and engagement exercises, their relative advantages and drawbacks and how to carry them out. If you are uncertain of how to proceed, get help from others who have done similar exercises before rather than waste time and effort on an exercise that is set up badly.

The section that follows lays out your pathways of choices. Start with the purpose – four main areas are given as examples.

► Improve information or communication for patients and the public to take account of their preferences.
► Make difficult decisions about treatment, funding or resources.
► Implement clinical governance.
► Assess and target needs within the limits of resources.

You may find that the purpose of *your* intended user involvement or public engagement exercise overlaps into several different areas; just look at each relevant section and choose methods that might suit more than one purpose or use a method from each. For each purpose, several specific objectives are listed but you might frame others more pertinent to your situation or that are more urgent for you to resolve. Several examples follow that describe typical topics that practices, PCGs and trusts often identify as problem areas or sources of friction between the services and NHS care that they provide and patients' and the public's perspectives of what they want or receive.

Suggestions for alternative methods you might select are given according to whether you are considering the user involvement or public engagement exercise from a population perspective – your practice, district or local community – or from the perspective of an identifiable patient group or individuals within that group – elderly people, those with disabilities, carers of those with dementia, etc. From there, the choice of methods is further subdivided into whether you want to 'interact' with the users or the public so that there is a two-way exchange of information or mainly want to 'receive' or to 'give' information. When you are considering how to involve the 'general public' or your whole 'patient population', at least one of your chosen methods will need to be a way of interacting with 'non-users' as well as 'users'; whilst if you intend to involve 'identifiable patient groups', they should be more straightforward to reach.

Don't forget, these methods are not a choice between one or another as any involvement or opinion exercise will be more valid if you obtain views and input from more than one source to minimise bias. So if you are considering an important topic and want wide-ranging views, choose two or three different methods, put the results together and compare your findings. For health needs assessment, you should think of involving the public and patients in the three approaches of gaining information about effectiveness, population data and services.

Don't cut corners because you do not have sufficient resources to undertake the user involvement exercise properly, so that you leave out essential stages like piloting questionnaires, using a convenience sample of people rather than a random sample or omitting the briefing session before one of the consensus methods. The reasons why you should keep to the standard scientific methods were explained in Chapter 4 and if you sacrifice best practice for expediency, you will devalue your exercise if your users are biased or too few and the outcome will be meaningless. If you do not have enough resources or skills, either wait until you have rectified the deficiency or select another method that you can afford or have the ability to undertake.

▼
Appropriate patient involvement.

How to do it – alternative pathways to user and public involvement

1 Purpose: To improve information or communication for patients or the general public and take account of their preferences

Possible specific objectives

- ▶ To find out what particular groups of patients want, if the quality of information and communication is good enough, if the information is accessible, if it is in a suitable format.
- ▶ To ascertain users' and non-users' views about the quality of information, the readability, contents, level of information of strategy documents or patient education materials.
- ▶ To assess whether particular patient groups have more problems with information or communication than others.
- ▶ To determine patients' expectations, preferences, needs – for access, range of services, personnel delivering care, responsiveness.
- ▶ To establish the preferences of lay people about the provision of health services and the management of medical conditions.
- ▶ To determine what levels of side effects or adverse consequences patients find acceptable when choosing to take up new or alternative treatments.
- ▶ To limit access to patients' medical records to the members of the multidisciplinary team that patients and the general public find acceptable.
- ▶ To find out whether patients are generally satisfied with the opportunities they have for consulting the health professionals of their choice.

Examples of topics you might consider

- ▶ Literature for patients undergoing tests. You might involve people in saying what they want, if the literature is accurate

Purpose: To improve information or communication for patients or the general public and take account of their preferences

Establish specific objectives

Agree priority topics to consider

Plan your involvement or consultation exercise

Consider selection of following example activities

If your target population is

practice population or local community

patient group, individual patients, carers

interactive process

Options:
- joint project or programme
- open meeting
- set up and operate website
- run a learning group
- journalist shadow health professional

interactive process

Options:
- workshop or seminar
- use patient participation group
- face-to-face interview survey
- discuss clinical management protocols

patients and public receive information

Options:
- trigger discussion on local radio
- compose and distribute newsletter
- run a roadshow
- run a healthline
- devise a tool to explain risks

patients receive information

Options:
- targeted letter to patients
- publish article in local press for people with specific health risks
- set up good practice library

patients and public give you information

Options:
- run focus groups
- questionnaire survey
- consult readers' panel
- study complaints log

patients give you information

Options:
- targeted telephone interviews
- lay person at training session
- visiting panel of appropriate patients
- 'suggestion slips' for patients
- audit information or communication

or detailed enough, if it is written in words with which patients are familiar, with a good balance between illustrations and text.

▸ The range of information for elderly people. You might find out how those who are hard of hearing, visually impaired or suffer from dementia currently fare and what they want in the way of written, pictorial, audiocassette, large print or video alternatives.

▸ The range and effectiveness of communication of health promotion messages to hard-to-reach groups, such as the homeless, gypsies/travellers, young men. Are messages reaching them in an appropriate way at the right time? Are the messages understood, do they make an impact and do changes in behaviour result?

▸ Strategy documents such as the Health Improvement Programme. You might involve people in defining priorities, planning how to present the messages, monitoring and implementing the plans or commenting on the contents of a draft version as to its relevance and readability.

▸ Health professionals' access to sources of evidence-based information and communication of that knowledge to patients; or direct access for lay people to similar sources.

▸ Alternative treatments for various cancers – patients' information needs, doctors' communication skills, the trust's, PCG's or practice's communication record.

▸ Patients' perceptions of risks or side effects of long-term treatments for various chronic illnesses.

▸ Patients' preferences for complementary and traditional therapies.

▸ Patients' satisfaction with their choice of gender, ethnicity or age of their usual or the latest doctor, nurse or therapist consulted.

▸ Ethnic differences such as different perceptions and expectations of health and illness.

Possible approach using one or several methods, depending on the purpose of the exercise and the available resources

If your target population is the whole practice population or local community

and you want to use an **interactive process for patients and the public to give and receive** information

- ► Operate joint working: joint managerial/lay/clinical input into a local project or programme.
- ► Hold an open meeting at the practice, PCG or trust with plenty of opportunities for discussion.
- ► Set up and operate your own website, advertising the availability of services, giving health messages and encouraging discussion or feedback; questions might be posed by the public for professionals to answer.
- ► Join a learning group (sometimes known as learner set, learning set, action learner set) of health and social care professionals and lay people set up as an educational activity where participants come to understand more about each others' constraints, capabilities, roles and responsibilities. The exercise will have most effect if the participants are relatively senior and can stimulate cultural changes in their own work setting, in response to their learning.
- ► Invite a journalist to spend time observing medical practice. Health professionals and the journalist will learn from each other and the learning will be subsequently passed onto the general lay readership.

or you want patients and the public to **receive** information from you

- ► Publish articles in the local press.
- ► Trigger a discussion topic on the local radio – send in a story, participate in a phone-in session, give an interview.
- ► Compose your own newsletter and distribute it to the local community or place it at public access points.

▶ Display posters in your waiting room which are informative and individualised for your practice or PCG or trust, describing topical matters.

▶ Run a roadshow with demonstrations of anything related to good information and communication systems or initiatives – perhaps in schools, community centres.

▶ Run a healthline at district level or dedicated phone-in time for general health information at the general practice level. Link or refer to NHS Direct or other national helplines as appropriate.

▶ Devise a tool (or use someone else's) to explain the risks of various treatment options to patients derived from published literature, comparing their risks with easily understandable risks in everyday life (for instance, being killed in a car accident).

<u>or you want patients and the public to **give** you information</u>

▶ Run focus groups involving representatives of particular groups of patients.

▶ Carry out a questionnaire survey:
   – general: e.g. in a newspaper or attached to a strategy document circulated to the public
   – targeted: as a postal survey or semistructured interviews, e.g. to special interest groups, user groups, key people
   – research study: for example, weighting of risks or views about alternative treatments. When results are disseminated in a journal, a wider population will be reached if the author writes short articles about the findings for the lay press.

▶ Consult a readers' panel: recruit a lay group to 'read' and give constructive feedback on draft business plans, strategy documents, etc.

▶ Study complaints: log verbal informal complaints and do an indepth review of relatively minor complaints and then act on the lessons by changing systems and practice.

If your target population is an identifiable patient group or individual patients or carers within that group

<u>and you want to use an</u> **interactive process for patients to give and receive** <u>information</u>

- ► Hold a workshop or seminar – do joint work in small groups. Rewrite information material for patients or delegate task to a lay writer.
- ► Use your patient participation group. Practice or trust staff might attend for an agenda item of joint interest to hear and explain each other's viewpoints.
- ► Carry out a face-to-face interview survey of a target population group in the course of routine work (for example, when visiting the housebound) by staff using a structured or semistructured interview schedule.
- ► Discuss clinical management protocols or guidelines with patients, such as via the Prodigy computerised decision support system, where associated education leaflets inform and enable patients to participate in the decision making.

<u>or you want patients to</u> **receive** <u>information from you</u>

- ► Send a targeted letter to patients with a particular problem, giving them an update of newly published evidence, for instance.
- ► Ask patients who have had particularly pertinent or 'ordinary' experiences of different treatment alternatives to write short accounts or tell their stories taped onto audiocassettes, to share with patients coming after them. Keep a database of such experienced patients prepared to telephone others newly presenting with the same problem, who need to speak to someone who has had a recent similar experience. Involve any trainees or students in the exercise.
- ► Set up a good practice library of patient educational materials from which to lend books, videos, CD-ROMs and audiocassettes to appropriate patients. Some commercial companies sponsor non-promotional material designed to

inform patients about the symptoms, signs and risks of their illness and encourage compliance with treatment.

▶ Publish articles in local press for lay readers with specific health risks such as smokers, those who are overweight or who are at risk of sexual diseases.

or you want patients to **give** you information

▶ Carry out a questionnaire survey. The method will depend on the characteristics of the patient group and if there are any social, cultural, language or ability limitations – use a postal survey or a telephone interview to targeted patients.

▶ Organise a training session with a lay person as one of the session's 'teachers' helping health professionals to understand the patient's perspective and why problems arise, such as non-compliance or disruptive behaviour.

▶ Set up an evaluation of a particular aspect of care or services that your practice, PCG or trust offers, by arranging for a visiting panel of appropriate patients or representatives of the public to assess the services with respect to the range, quality or difficulties of access.

▶ Attach 'suggestion slips' to repeat prescriptions or appointment letters of patients with particular conditions inviting their input about anything related to their care or specifically enquiring about an aspect of the service.

▶ Undertake an audit of an important aspect of the quality of information or communication. Involve lay people in setting the criteria and standards, reviewing performance compared to standards, discussing the changes.

▶ Run focus groups of patients with a particular experience. But beware members of users' groups who have become too polished at relaying their histories, for whom too much time has elapsed since the relevant experience for them to remember clearly the emotions and thoughts they had at the time.

2 Purpose: To make difficult decisions about treatment, funding or resources

Possible specific objectives

▶ To gain people's views about how decisions about rationing or prioritising services or treatments should be made, who should be involved and when.

▶ To review what factors should be considered when prioritising a health problem as regards the allocation of resources.

▶ To centralise services and reduce peripheral facilities.

▶ To take an overview about whether resources are allocated according to need between health and social care sectors or between health and education sectors.

▶ To look at reducing costs by using less skilled staff for the aspect of care under consideration; and if the skill mix is changed, to determine whether less skilled staff do actually cost less in the long run.

▶ To help patients share in decision making about alternative treatment options in informed and meaningful ways.

▶ To find out what services patients or the general public think the NHS should provide for particular groups of people.

▶ To determine people's views before a new procedure is brought in, to understand their information needs and afterwards to learn from their experiences.

Examples of topics you might consider

▶ Agree local criteria for funding non-life-saving medical treatments such as fertility treatments.

▶ Substitute nurses for doctors, assistants for qualified therapists, counsellors for psychologists to provide healthcare services.

▶ Review funding arrangements, responsibilities of staff in health and social care organisations for bathing elderly people at home or providing aids for people with disabilities.

Purpose: To make difficult decisions about treatment, funding or resources

Establish specific objectives

Agree priority topics to consider

Plan your involvement or consultation exercise

Consider selection of following example activities

If your target population is

practice population or local community

patient group, individual patients, carers

interactive process

Options:
- ► consensus development conference
- ► Delphi study
- ► public meeting
- ► citizens' jury
- ► lay representative on board as conduit
- ► presentations to groups, discussions
- ► talk with Community Health Council
- ► public notices
- ► prize winning competition
- ► advertise board meetings well to public

interactive process

Options:
- ► lend videos
- ► sit in on users' group as observer
- ► run nominal groups
- ► give presentations to users' groups
- ► invite comments on draft plan
- ► involve users in evaluating service
- ► patient record diaries
- ► hand-held patients' records

patients and public receive information

Options:
- ► hold discussion on local radio
- ► hold roadshow
- ► health information booklet to households
- ► work through voluntary organisations to hard-to-reach groups

patients receive information

Options:
- ► particular patient/group give lay perspective
- ► create library of resources for patients
- ► lay people act as advocates
- ► organise co-ordinated cascade
- ► use others' communication system
- ► start correspondence in local newspaper

patients and public give you information

Options:
- ► set up and use standing panel
- ► one-off opinion poll
- ► focus groups
- ► semistructured interviews
- ► neighbourhood forums
- ► rapid appraisal initiative

patients give you information

Options:
- ► community development project
- ► focus groups
- ► nominal groups
- ► face-to-face interviews
- ► feedback or evaluation slips

▶ Agree if and what social, age, lifestyle and prognostic criteria might be applied to limit people's entitlement to expensive treatments such as kidney transplantation or cardiac surgery.

▶ The extent of patients' choice with respect to referral for a medical opinion or treatment outside the district.

▶ How investment decisions should be made with regard to reducing waiting lists for treatment; weighing resources for the treatment of potentially life-threatening against treatment for incapacitating but non-life-threatening conditions.

▶ Gauging views about whether people with acute eye problems would consult an optometrist instead of a GP or the A&E department and if such a service is acceptable, how should access be arranged and should users pay a fee?

▶ Patients' and the public's views on whether complementary therapy should be available as part of NHS treatment and if so, which therapies should be included?

▶ Changing surgery opening hours.

Possible approach using one or several methods, depending on the purpose of the exercise and the available resources

If your target population is the whole practice population or local community

and you want to use an **interactive process for patients and the public to give and receive** information and opinions about making difficult decisions

▶ Run a consensus development conference with a mix of professionals and lay people.

▶ Consider a Delphi study of key leaders in the locality.

▶ See if your overarching organisation – the PCG, trust, health authority, region or central NHS Executive – will help look after your interests by organising a co-ordinated and equitable approach to the difficult decision. They will have more resources for obtaining a wider cross-section of views and exchanging information with the local community.

- ▶ Organise a public consultation meeting.
- ▶ Set up a citizens' jury, briefed well, to consider the issues and prioritise different action plans.
- ▶ Ask the lay representative(s) on the PCG or trust board to serve as a conduit for a two-way exchange of information with their networks with the public.
- ▶ Make presentations to groups with particular interests or responsibilities for the subject in question, with plenary discussions.
- ▶ Feedback and exchange information with the Community Health Council, who may conduct their own consultation.
- ▶ Compose public notices or published articles setting out the issues and proposals and inviting comments, either in answer to structured questions or as free comments.
- ▶ Run a competition with a small prize for people who send in the best name for the planned new venture – that should attract more people's notice – and give you an opportunity to explain the rationale for the planned changes and invite comments at the same time.
- ▶ Advertise the board meetings of the PCG or trust well to the public. Make the lay or staff audience feel welcome and invite them to participate.

or you want patients and the public to **receive** information and opinions about making difficult decisions

- ▶ Interest the media in holding a discussion on the topic on the local radio; participate in a phone-in session, contribute to a debate and give an interview to explain the issues.
- ▶ Hold a roadshow, presenting the issues and describing the alternatives. Give anonymised examples from real life so that people can understand how the limited resources affect people's way of life or well-being.
- ▶ Deliver health information booklet to all households advising about appropriate action to take for medical problems, using patients' representatives to help with the distribution.
- ▶ Use voluntary organisations and their contacts and networks to communicate with hard-to-reach groups of the population.

► Submit articles to the press. Try and interest the press sufficiently so that they send a photographer along; the picture will capture people's attention more effectively than text.

or you want patients and the public to **give** you information and opinions about making difficult decisions

► Set up and use a standing panel or consult the population using someone else's panel. Has your local authority set up a standing citizens' panel that you could tag onto for health matters?

► Commission opinion poll by market research company in the street or by telephone.

► Run focus groups but you might want to avoid patients or their families directly suffering as a result of limited resources to treat the condition or circumstances at issue, if you want considered opinions as opposed to an emotional wrangle.

► Look for other models outside the health service where the public inform difficult decision making and see if their approach is feasible for you.

► Carry out semistructured interviews with senior members of community, key opinion leaders, etc.

► Contact neighbourhood forums and ask them to debate the issues at their next meetings. Make a regular arrangement with a local forum so that you can each select an item for the other's agenda and feedback views.

► Organise a rapid appraisal initiative. Use a mix of community development approaches for a snapshot of all the different types of information known about the issue in a particular community and talk to key people to find out their views.

► Carry out a literature search or ask around; has anyone tried what you are proposing elsewhere? Phone up contacts and discuss the pros and cons of how their new services or changes are working out. Learn from them and generalise their experiences to your situation if you can.

If your target population is an identifiable patient group or individual patients or carers within that group

and you want to use an **interactive process for patients to give and receive** information and opinions about making difficult decisions

▶ Lend a video to an individual patient with a serious condition for which a difficult decision must be made. Or find other educational material (see Appendix 1) that is appropriate to what they want and need to know about their options. Once they are well informed, you will be able to share the decision making in a more meaningful way.

▶ Sit in on a users' group as an observer; it will soon become an interactive exchange as the users make the most of the opportunity to ask you questions and you hear their concerns and can discuss decision making about difficult issues!

▶ Run nominal groups with interested organisations.

▶ Organise presentations to particular users' groups by someone at the centre with a grasp of the issues, followed by an interactive discussion. Explain advantages of the planned changes over the current system.

▶ Send a draft plan to a voluntary group or a patients' group and ask for comments or ask them to plan out how they will implement your proposal.

▶ Set up a pilot project and involve users and staff in evaluating how well the new service or arrangements work at every stage. Be prepared to revise or discard such an initiative if it is rated as unpopular or ineffective.

▶ Use record diaries to allow patients to log the frequency and magnitude of their symptoms prospectively over a month or longer; this should trigger the advice and information they really want from the doctor, nurse or therapist at the next consultation.

▶ Introduce and evaluate the use of patient-held records for a chronic medical condition. Such records should improve shared decision making as the patient is kept up to date with their current management, enabling them to reflect on future options before the associated decision has to be taken.

or you want patients to **receive** information and opinions about making difficult decisions

- ▶ Arrange for others who have suffered the same problem to talk to a particular patient or patient group to give their lay perspectives of the alternatives available.

- ▶ Arrange for one or more carers who have made difficult decisions in the past to talk to a carer or group of carers who are having problems with the person they are caring for. Join the discussion and learn at first hand how people make such decisions so that you have more understanding in the future.

- ▶ Create a practice, PCG or trust library of resources where patients can borrow appropriate books, tapes and videos to inform them about the issues to consider when making their own critical decisions.

- ▶ Recruit lay people to act as advocates for patients who are fazed by authority or intellectually unable to take their own decisions, to befriend such patients and help them make rational decisions about treatment options.

- ▶ Organise a co-ordinated cascade system for passing on information, via staff or representatives of patients' groups.

- ▶ Display warning notices about any planned changes several weeks before the changes occur to get people familiar with the new systems; write a simple information leaflet describing the planned changes and giving a timetable of events.

- ▶ Piggyback onto some other organisation's communication system. Next time they are circulating particular patients or groups, add a memo or letter from you to their correspondence.

- ▶ Write a letter to the local newspaper – many individual patients will read that. Ask people to tell others about the issues in your letter and contact you if they wish.

or you want patients to **give** you information and opinions about making difficult decisions

- ▶ Use a community development project that is already established to gather information about the issue. Ask appropriate people at your local health promotion department or city council what community development is taking place.

▶ Ask a patient who has made a difficult decision about treatment options how they might have been helped more or been better informed.

▶ Run focus groups, perhaps of carers or patients with a condition relevant to the planned change.

▶ Organise nominal groups of people involved in providing the changes – health and social care professionals – and those receiving care or representing those that do – lay people, as unidisciplinary or mixed groups.

▶ Carry out face-to-face interviews or make a simple enquiry of the individual patients or carers most likely to be affected. Interviews might be carried out by able lay people from a voluntary organisation, for example.

▶ Give out or administer simple feedback or evaluation slips for people using the pilot or current service that you plan to change, inviting views about current standards, wants and needs. Try to arrange the enquiry so that responses are anonymous and non-identifable to encourage people to give honest replies.

3 Purpose: To implement clinical governance

Background

Clinical governance has been defined as 'a framework through which NHS organisations are accountable for continuously improving the quality of their services, safeguarding high standards by creating an environment in which excellence in clinical care will flourish'.[1]

Possible specific objectives

▶ To monitor or improve the quality of selected examples of clinical care or aspects of services.

Purpose: To implement clinical governance

Establish specific objectives

Agree priority topics to consider

Plan your involvement or consultation exercise

Consider selection of following example activities

If your target population is

practice population or local community

patient group, individual patients, carers

interactive process

Options:
- ▶ run seminar for users and carers
- ▶ standing panel
- ▶ create Patient's Charter
- ▶ bulletin board on website

interactive process

Options:
- ▶ presentation to patients' groups
- ▶ patient participation group comment
- ▶ register for higher award of quality
- ▶ design information leaflets for particular groups

patients receive information

patients and public receive information

Options:
- ▶ newsletter describing standards
- ▶ present comparative information about prescribing patterns
- ▶ submit article to local press

Options:
- ▶ information leaflets for particular groups
- ▶ patients' 'mini-charters' of best practice
- ▶ summary of news to patients, carers

patients give you information

patients and public give you information

Options:
- ▶ audit telephone access
- ▶ visiting panel of lay people
- ▶ track numbers of patients
- ▶ focus groups

Options:
- ▶ disabled person in wheelchair looks round your premises
- ▶ focus group of users
- ▶ focus groups of carers
- ▶ lay input into training sessions

- To find out whether there are any problems with access to care for different patient groups and where access might be improved.
- To assess the quality of care of a medical condition with regard to diagnosis, investigation, clinical and organisational management.
- To determine the quality of interpersonal relationships between all the health professionals and support staff with whom particular patients come into contact.
- To look from the patient's perspective at whether NHS staff have appropriate skills, attitudes and knowledge with respect to providing healthcare for specific medical conditions.
- To explore whether doctors and nurses explain evidence-based or best practice of clinical management in ways that convince patients so that they comply with recommended treatment regimes.

Examples of topics you might consider

- Prescribing patterns and adherence to agreed prescribing policies.
- Access for the disabled to premises and toilets and when climbing up onto an examination couch.
- Conforming of practitioners' chronic disease management to agreed evidence-based management protocols.
- Quality of consultation from patient's point of view – health professional listens, explains, appears technically competent, gives clear advice and instructions, shares decisions.
- Risk management policies exist and are applied, for example in the rapid response to patients presenting with life-threatening emergencies.
- An objective educational assessment of clinical and support staff's capabilities to undertake patient information or public involvement activities in a meaningful way. Design an educational programme to rectify gaps in knowledge, attitudes and skills.

Possible approach using one or several methods, depending on the purpose of the exercise and the available resources

If your target population is the whole practice population or local community

and you want to use an **interactive process for patients and the public to give and receive** input about the implementing of clinical governance

▶ Run a seminar for users and carers and representatives of voluntary organisations to explain the meaning, issues and implications of clinical governance; invite informed patients and the public to participate in a second seminar with clinicians and managers to agree priorities for a clinical governance development programme.

▶ Use a standing panel to establish concerns and priorities about the quality of care and services to be addressed under the clinical governance umbrella.

▶ Create a Patient's Charter after preliminary qualitative work with patients' groups to establish what rights all, or a particular group of, patients can realistically expect and what responsibilities those patients should assume. Monitor the extent to which the Charter standards are met, by involving a visiting lay panel or the lay representative on the PCG or trust board, the Community Health Council or other patients' representatives.

▶ Advertise a bulletin board on your website for news and discussion about standards of healthcare in the practice or trust.

or you want patients and the public to **receive** feedback or news about the implementing of clinical governance

▶ Publish a newsletter describing the standards of care your practice, PCG or trust aspires to or reached recently.

▶ Present identifiable comparative information about prescribing patterns at a public board meeting with the agreement of the clinicians (*note*: this idea might be better placed in the 'interactive' category as you are bound to trigger a lot of discussion and debate by releasing such sensitive information).

▶ Submit an article to the local press about the success of a recent initiative or new services that have been established.

or you want patients and the public to **give** you input about the implementing of clinical governance

▶ Audit telephone access: find out from the telephone company what proportion of callers find the line engaged at peak periods. Ask patients to comment on whether the standards of telephone access achieved are acceptable.

▶ Ask a visiting panel of lay people to comment on access to your premises, then invite them to reassess the situation after you have made improvements.

▶ Track a specific number of patients with the medical problems you are studying and ask them to report prospectively on their experiences at stages in their care pathway from primary care to secondary care and the parallel treatment by staff in both sectors. Ask about various aspects of the quality of care they received. Discuss the results at a management meeting.

▶ Organise focus groups – of patients with same condition.

If your target population is an identifiable patient group or individual patients or carers within that group

and you want to use an **interactive process with patients, carers and non-users to give and receive** input about implementing clinical governance

▶ Make a presentation to particular patients' groups by GPs, nurses or managers, followed by opportunities for discussion and exchange of views.

▶ Invite your patient participation group to comment on your practice developmental plan in detail; arrange equal numbers of lay people and key members of the practice team.

▼

Lay input into training sessions can be valuable.

Facilitate interactive exchange where people are free to give constructive comments without fear.

► Register for a higher award of quality,[2] such as Investors in People, the British Standards Institute ISO 9000 scheme, the Charter Mark scheme or the Royal College of General Practitioners' Fellowship by Assessment; the interaction that results will not only include review and discussion of the quality and purpose of staff training but will require two-way interchanges with users, carers and non-users on audit, effectiveness and all aspects of the organisation.

► Design information leaflets for particular groups with the help of some of their members to give essential information; for example, leaflets to catch adolescents' attention about the availability of emergency contraception will benefit from a youngster advising on the content and presentation. Attaching a comment slip with freepost address on the reverse side might attract suggestions for meeting their needs – time, place, personnel, etc.

or you want patients, carers and non-users to **receive** input about implementing clinical governance from you

► Design information leaflets for particular groups as for the interactive exchange above but without feedback slips; target elderly people, youngsters.

► Give patients 'mini-charters' listing best practice in the management of their chronic conditions so that they can compare the management they receive against this information. The information about best practice might come from decision support systems such as Prodigy computer software, self-help associations, an Internet site or be derived from the National Institute of Clinical Effectiveness (NICE) guidelines or the National Service Frameworks (NSF).

► Send a short summary of news about your activities that come under the clinical governance umbrella to secretaries of key patient, carer and professional groups or organisations from other sectors such as schools or day centres; keep them informed about your improvement programme and how they might get involved. Include groups and their representatives whom you have never thought of writing to before but who contribute to the provision of healthcare locally. This should have the additional benefit of encouraging networking and joint working and reducing duplication of initiatives.

or you want patients, carers and non-users to **give** you input about implementing clinical governance

► Take a disabled person in a wheelchair round your premises into every part where you would expect an able-bodied patient to have access. Ask them to point out the difficulties and impossibilities and give you ideas on ways to overcome the problems.

► Set up a focus group of users: for example, to debate access and availability of services or discuss the usual reception they experience from staff.

► Run a focus group with carers: for example, to debate the availability of home visits, response to out-of-hours requests for medical care, provision of equipment and aids, continuity of care from multidisciplinary team.

► Arrange lay input into training sessions of support staff and clinicians, to encourage training to be relevant to patients' needs.

4 Purpose: To assess and target needs appropriately within the limits of resources

Background

The ten steps of health needs assessment are:

1 understand your population
2 identify the incidence and prevalence of the condition or problem
3 calculate the expected number of cases
4 measure service utilisation
5 calculate unmet needs
6 review effectiveness of interventions
7 seek population's views
8 find out professionals' views
9 agree priorities
10 define interventions and healthcare programmes.[3,4]

That is, health needs assessment encompasses the potential to benefit from care (need), expressed desire for services (demand) and services that are actually provided in relation to need or demand (supply). Health needs assessment includes epidemiological, comparative, corporate and qualitative approaches with 'macro' population or 'micro' patient-based perspectives.

Possible specific objectives

► To draw up a profile of the local population, including the structure, environment, lifestyles, culture and religions, measures of disease and disability.

Purpose: To assess and target needs appropriately within the limits of resources

Establish specific objectives

Agree priority topics to consider

Plan your involvement or consultation exercise

Consider selection of following example activities

If your target population is

practice population or local community

patient group, individual patients, carers

interactive process

Options:
► community development approach
► rapid appraisal
► consensus methods: nominal group, consensus development conference, Delphi survey
► questionnaire survey of public
► weekly column in local newspaper
► website
► attend community-based decision-making bodies
► via lay representative(s) on NHS boards
► locally based information project

interactive process

Options:
► patient participation group
► research and development or audit project
► meet and confer with various special interest groups

patients receive information

Options:
► write in local newsletters to patient groups
► patient representative observes need or best practice
► contact particular population group for informal 'chat'
► employ support worker as link to patient group

patients and public receive information

Options:
► newspaper articles
► local radio: health promotion
► targeted health promotion for hard-to-reach groups

patients give you information

Options:
► focus groups
► interviews
► comment slips for patients
► undertake library search
► health parliament

patients and public give you information

Options:
► questionnaire survey
► poster campaign
► comment slips for the public

► To identify the needs of the whole community, particular patient groups or individual patients that are not (fully) addressed by current services.

► To contain demand for services at levels commensurate with current resources.

► To determine whether any particular patient groups are discriminated against or in other ways disadvantaged by current ways of planning and delivering NHS services.

► To look at the quality of care according to several or all of Maxwell's dimensions of quality, namely: efficiency and economy, effectiveness (for individual patients), relevance to need (for the whole community), social acceptability, equity and access to services, with respect to all of the district population or subsections of the community.[5]

► To consider fair ways of weighting resources between different practices or subgroups of the population in a PCG population, for various aspects of patient care.

► To compare the different approaches of social services, the health authority, a PCG and community nurses to health needs assessments and determine whether any way is more effective than another for reaching and involving particular patient populations.

► To determine the most effective interventions for particular conditions.

Examples of topics you might consider

► Out-of-hours care: assess the quality of provision of out-of-hours medical care at trust, PCG or practice levels or from the health authority perspective across the district.

► Any of the objectives for patients with particular characteristics such as adolescents, young mothers, elderly people, employed people whose working hours restrict their access to medical care, people without a car or telephone.

► Any of the objectives for people with particular needs such as those with a learning disability, people with severe mental health problems, the homeless, deprived communities such as those that live in remote rural areas or the inner cities.

▶ The needs of various ethnic groups with respect to known ethnic differences such as different disease patterns, different cultures, racism and discrimination, lack of involvement in planning and organisation of their health services.[3]

▶ Assessment of needs and provision of services for house-bound people: carers who find difficulty leaving their charges, people with profound disabilities, those who are terminally ill.

Possible approach using one or several methods, depending on the purpose of the exercise and the available resources

If your target population is the whole practice population or local community

and you want to use an **interactive process for patients and the public to give and receive** information and advice about assessing and targeting patients' or the general public's needs

▶ Adopt a community development approach: co-ordinate or work through the community development workers, health promotion facilitators, health visitors, social workers, employees and volunteers in the non-statutory sector who are already in post.

▶ Use rapid appraisal: involve health professionals, social workers and others to encourage ownership of findings and eventual solutions. Hold further discussions with the general public when the findings are published whilst evolving and deciding on the best solutions.

▶ Employ a consensus method: nominal group, consensus development conference, Delphi survey – depending on how wide ranging the topic is.

▶ Undertake a questionnaire survey of the general public: place in a newspaper or attach to a strategy document such as the Health Improvement Programme (this is in a *give and receive* category because such a questionnaire would be attached to a newspaper article or document describing the plans and discussing the issues).

▶ Speak in a local radio discussion programme or phone-in.

▶ Contribute a weekly column in local newspaper to which experts contribute to readers' comments and suggestions.

▶ Establish a website: interactive discussion group for lay and health professionals.

▶ Key representatives of health authority, PCG, trust or general practices become members of or attend community-based decision-making bodies in local politics, education, local authority, etc.

▶ Lay representative(s) or non-executive director(s) of trust, health authority, PCG interact with the boards of these organisations and the constituency and lay organisations they represent.

▶ Use a district or subdistrict-based information project to pool data held by the different organisations: for instance, the project might look at establishing the minimum amount of information required, and from which sources that information might be obtained, in order to carry out a health needs assessment for the topic in question. The sources will be diverse and are bound to include lay and health and social care organisations if a wide enough approach is taken. A shared lay–health professional lead will enable joint working to occur in a meaningful way.

or you want patients and the public to **receive** information about assessing and targeting patients' or the general public's needs from you

▶ Write for the local newspaper giving information directed at particular groups or informing the general public about particular groups.

▶ Local radio: health club type of health promotion pro-gramme such as 'smokebusters' aimed at engaging young people in stopping smoking.

▶ Target health promotion at hard-to-reach groups, through representatives of those groups acting as facilitators or different conduits such as touring theatre groups in schools performing a play highlighting health messages.

<u>or you want patients and the public to</u> **give** <u>you information and advice about assessing and targeting patients' or the general public's needs</u>

- ▸ Undertake a questionnaire survey: for example, a random selection from the local electoral register.
- ▸ Begin a poster campaign inviting people to write or phone in with comments and suggestions.
- ▸ Leave comment slips at public access points, day centres, pharmacies or playgroups, for instance, to reach people not using general practices.

If your target population is an identifiable patient group or individual patients or carers within that group

<u>and you want to use an</u> **interactive process for patients to give and receive** <u>information and advice about assessing and targeting patients' or the general public's needs</u>

- ▸ Meet with a patient participation group to discuss the issues, for them to act as go-betweens with the constituencies they represent, relaying concerns and ideas.
- ▸ Carry out a relevant research and development or audit project at local level in which health professionals and lay people or patients take active parts.
- ▸ Meet and confer with various special interest groups.

<u>or you want patients to</u> **receive** <u>information and advice about assessing and targeting patients' or the general public's needs from you</u>

- ▸ Contribute articles to local newsletters sent out to particular patient groups, for example users' group or carers' group newsletters, giving information known about needs and any mismatch in services.
- ▸ Welcome a representative of a particular group to the trust or general practice and arrange for them to observe evidence

of need or best practice at first hand, to relay back to the populations they represent.

► Work through a friendly contact from a particular population group and get them to introduce you to their group for you to chat to them about the issues or employ a support worker as a link with that group of carers, the homeless, etc.

or you want patients to **give** you information and advice about assessing and targeting patients' or the general public's needs

► Run focus groups of hard-to-reach groups, user groups.
► Carry out interviews with consecutive individual patients who match the category under enquiry to find out more about their recent experiences, perceived needs (according to the patient) and observed needs (according to the health professional or an independent source). You might recruit subjects through the 'snowballing' technique whereby members of hard-to-reach groups who are known are asked to recruit others for the survey. You might use semistructured or unstructured interviews to encourage personal accounts.
► Give comment slips to people using the current service under review.
► Undertake a library search: there is a great deal of published literature about the needs of different population groups. Précis the material relevant to your locality.
► Set up a health parliament of a particular age group; for example, elected members of young people's groups and the education sector or older people from diverse groups with an older membership (sport, clubs, day centres, etc).

Approximate costings of alternative methods of informing patients, involving patients and the public in planning and delivering healthcare

The costings are difficult to quantify because the exact budget will depend on the size of the exercise, how difficult it is to reach the target population, how skilled the personnel involved are or need to be, whether health professionals and others are incorporating the extra work into their daily activities and what the consequent opportunity costs are. Although the budgets look substantial when priced up in these approximate ways, the real costs of *not* involving the public or patients in meaningful ways could be very high, in terms of providing healthcare and services that are not in tune with what patients and the public need or will use or in human misery if patients are ill informed and poorly served.

Providing better education and information

- Patient education leaflets, books, videos, audiocassettes: some non-promotional ones may be free from pharmaceutical companies or produced at subsidised rates. A practice library with sufficient material to lend to patients on a variety of conditions will cost at least £2000 with ongoing replacement costs if patients do not return the goods.
- One-off presentation and subsequent discussion: will take at least four hours of a health professional's time if preparation, travel and attendance are included.
- Writing an article for a local newspaper or a newsletter: depends on your skill and experience but it will probably take most health professionals about three hours to write and polish a 300-word article if they are unused to writing.
- Participate in a phone-in on radio: the time taken will include travel to and from the recording studio unless you speak on an outside phone line as a contributor to the discussion, rather than receiving and answering all the calls. Also remember to include the preparation time, as you would be unwise to speak on the radio without having reflected upon key points you want to bring up and having the basic facts or statistics to hand. Additional costs would be employing a member of staff on public relations duties if that was necessary to set up media and press contacts.

► Communication skills training: a training session should be as interactive as possible in a small group and may involve being videoed. This may entail a relatively expensive attendance fee unless the course is provided free as part of local professional training.

► Make your own video: your local university might have the facilities for you to make your own videos in a professional studio. The charges will depend on your local situation but might be about £1000 plus the costs of the videotapes.

► Your own web page: you can create your own web page through generally available software from an Internet access provider or pay someone with the know-how to design an attractive website for you and update it.

Exchanging and obtaining information

► Focus group: staff time includes the facilitator's and observer's time for about two hours preparation, two hours attendance and several hours to write up a report, plus the secretarial time of about eight hours to transcribe a one-hour audiocassette tape and time to arrange the meeting. In addition, there are the costs of hospitality (maybe as much as a meal in a hotel), reimbursement of the participants' travel expenses and fees if applicable. The first time you run a focus group, you may need to buy a good tape-recording machine that picks up conversation from several metres away and a transcribing machine for the secretary. Costs for staff time alone might be £100–300 per focus group, depending on the seniority of staff employed on the exercise and the amount of preparation and writing-up time involved.

► A questionnaire survey or Delphi survey: one healthcare survey of 250 people, where the questionnaire was given out to respondents in person and returned in freepost envelopes, took 121 hours of a researcher's time from designing the questionnaires to writing up the report but excluding the preparatory stage of carrying out a literature search and gathering qualitative information by interviewing people typical of the population to which the questionnaire would later be despatched.[6] Other costs included the stationery, photocopying, postage, secretarial help with coding returned questionnaires (in the case cited, it took 27 hours) and a statistician's time for analysis (in this case, it took ten hours) and use of the computer hardware and statistical software. Thus, if an experienced research assistant with interviewing skills, earning around £10 an hour, was employed on the survey, the total costs might be around £2000 without taking account of overheads and expenses. As a guide for those who need to buy 'names' and their contact details from a population database for a survey, a typical cost might be in the region of £200 per 1000 randomly selected details from the electoral register of Stoke-on-Trent city (1999 prices).

▶ Undertaking an interview study: each interview of an hour probably takes about eight hours of the interviewer's time which includes preparing for the interview, making the appointment, travel, doing the interview, writing it up, with considerable extra time if the interviews are being taped and transcribed. Thus, a researcher earning around £10 an hour who spends about 400 hours carrying out about 30 interviews and extra time transcribing audiotapes will cost about £4000 plus travel costs and other survey costs such as statistical help if required.

▶ Rapid appraisal: in the project described on pp. 61–2, the GP author, a health visitor colleague and two others spent around 48 hours each actively gathering information. There would be additional costs for preparing and writing up the interviews; the published report indicated that 25 or so interviews might be sufficient. If a researcher was used instead of health professionals and the researcher's time was priced at £10 per hour as in the other examples, the cost would be about £3200 for 25 transcribed interviews and, with around £2000 for gathering data from other sources, travel expenses and writing the final report, the minimum research bill would be about £5600 without overheads. There would be additional costs for the health professionals and other key figures to read, reflect on and discuss the findings and make plans to address the needs.

▶ Community development: programmes often have a community development worker employed as a full-time project worker on a temporary contract. The size and purpose of the project will dictate how long the community worker is employed for, and thus the costs, but such work often takes 1–2 years to gain the trust of the local community, build up networks, plan interventions and put them into place.

▶ Opinion poll: depends on the number of people being questioned and how accessible they are. If a market research company carries out such a survey, they charge commercial rates. You can get an idea of their charging rates from knowing that 'market research or similar organisations ... charged approximately £4000 to £6000 (for recruiting jurors to a citizens' jury), a fee which included two group discussions with members of the public'.[8]

▶ Citizens' jury: typical costs are quoted as being around £16 000 plus considerable staff time,[8] up to £30 000.[9]

▶ Neighbourhood forum, patient participation group, user group: members are volunteers. Thus the expenses will be those of organising the event, possibly reimbursing travel expenses, providing light refreshments, taking minutes and writing and distributing any ensuing report or newsletter. Such a forum or group probably costs the NHS less than £100 a meeting, the comparatively low cost being because participants give their time without charge.

▶ Standing panel or health parliament: participants are volunteers. The costs include setting up the panel and recruiting members, organising the panel and obtaining new members to replace those whose term has expired or who have left the panel, communicating with the panel and enclosing a free-post means of response. If the clerical time required was about 12 hours a week and 500 participants took part in four polls a year, the costs might be around £6000 per year, plus overheads. However, one costing described by Staffordshire County Council for a citizens' panel is £40 000 in the first year and £19 000 for the next two years[10] for four surveys a year organised by the London-based opinion poll firm MORI. The panel will start with 200 citizens to which local borough councils can join in, adding their own questions and the numbers of residents involved.

▶ Regular staff undertaking brief structured interviews of individual patients as part of consultations: these would have to be brief if they are to be incorporated into staff's normal work. Costs would be in training staff in interview skills and some clerical time to collate results.

▶ Nominal group: the organiser and facilitator might spend ten hours between them planning, organising and attending the group meeting and writing up a relatively brief report. The participants would probably be attending as part of their everyday work or as volunteers. Additional costs would be for the venue and hospitality and reimbursement of travel expenses. If the organising staff time was priced at £10 an hour as in the other examples given, the costs of running a nominal group would be less than £200 without taking account of the opportunity costs of any staff or lay participants.

References

1 Department of Health (1998) *A First Class Service: Quality in the New NHS*. Department of Health, London.

2 Roland M, Holden J, Campbell S (1999) *Quality Assessment for General Practice: Supporting Clinical Governance in Primary Care Groups*. National Primary Care Research and Development Centre, University of Manchester.

3 Rawaf S, Bahl V (1998) *Assessing Health Needs of People from Minority Ethnic Groups*. Royal College of Physicians, London.

4 Harris A (ed) (1997) *Needs to Know: A Guide to Needs Assessment for Primary Care*. Churchill Livingstone, London.

5 Maxwell RJ (1984) Quality assessment in health. *BMJ*. **288**: 1470–2.

6 Chambers R (1993) How long did it take and what did it cost? A study of the time and costs involved in carrying out a research survey. *Postgrad Educ Gen Pract.* **4**: 37–40.

7 Murray SA, Tapson J, Turnbull L *et al.* (1994) Listening to local voices: adapting rapid appraisal to assess health and social needs in general practice. *BMJ.* **308**: 698–700.

8 McIver S (1998) *Healthy Debate? An Independent Evaluation of Citizens' Juries in Health Settings.* King's Fund, London.

9 Coote A (1999) Citizens' jury: a forum for health debate (editorial). *Update.* **18 March**: 485.

10 Manson R (1999) Families' chance to have say on council services. *The Sentinel.* **April 21**: 9.

CHAPTER 6

Giving patients and the public more information

Informing patients and carers better

Patients ought to know what is wrong with them, what is likely to happen to them and what treatment they require. Why should anyone allow someone else to make decisions for them about their health? The better the information patients receive, the better able they are to participate in decision making about their own clinical management and make informed choices about different alternatives of care. There is some evidence that well-informed patients who actively share in making decisions about treatment have more favourable health outcomes – for instance, improved control of blood sugar levels in the care of diabetics.[1] Giving patients more information has been associated with greater patient satisfaction,[2] as the study described in the box below shows.

Giving patients more information leads to increased patient satisfaction, better compliance and better recall and understanding of medical conditions[2]

A review of 41 research studies on this topic showed that there was a correlation between patients receiving good information at a healthcare consultation and:

► greater patient satisfaction

continued

continued

▶ better compliance as measured by keeping future appointments or complying with their care regimen
▶ greater recall of how much information given at a previous consultation was remembered at a later visit
▶ greater understanding of the medical condition after the consultation
▶ patients being female

and trends rather than correlations for whether patients received good information and their having higher levels of social class, income and educational attainment.

Patient satisfaction was increased according to the extent of communication in the consultation as rated by either the length of consultation in minutes or numbers of practitioner/patient utterances.

Some doctors and nurses are reluctant to share information, thinking that it may encourage patients to make more demands and so increase their workloads. Others fear that parting with information may render them more vulnerable to criticism if patients are in a better position to judge health professionals' performance and the standards of treatment they receive.

There may be a mismatch between what information doctors and other health professionals consider to be important and what patients think. The top three suggestions for a revamped Patient's Charter that members of the Patients' Association would like to see are that:

▶ general practitioners should have to give patients clear reasons before striking them off their lists
▶ patients should have access to data on their doctors' performance
▶ patients should be in charge of their own medical notes.

Patient empowerment.

In a survey commissioned by Which, patients prioritised five areas of practice for improvement significantly more often than GPs did.[3] These were:

▶ the need to reduce time spent waiting – in the waiting room or for an appointment
▶ GPs' attention to what patients say
▶ GPs' explanations to patients

▶ convenience of surgery hours
▶ the extent to which GPs involve patients in treatment choices.

Another study of people's priorities with respect to general practice care found that patients the world over had many similar views, mostly focused on the quality of communication with their doctors.[4] The majority of respondents put most emphasis on being able to spend time talking with their general practitioners, doctors telling patients all they want to know about their illnesses, making patients feel free to talk about their problems and confidentiality of information about patients.

If carers are better informed and their contribution to the overall care of the dependent person is acknowledged, welcomed and respected by health professionals, they should be able to take more responsibility and be more likely to seek professional help appropriately.

Giving patients more and better information is more complex than it may seem at first sight. Doctors and other health professionals are more likely to favour some patients with information above others. A study undertaken in America showed that well-educated, middle-aged female patients were the group most likely to receive good information at their healthcare consultations.[5] The findings are reported in the box below.

Patients' characteristics can compromise the effectiveness of interpersonal care

Doctors are less likely to involve certain types of patients in making decisions about their healthcare than others.[5] Patients who seem to have the least interaction with their doctors are:

▶ elderly people aged 75 years and older
▶ young adults, aged under 30
▶ patients who did not attend further education
▶ patients from minority groups
▶ male patients.

continued

continued

Men were less likely to participate in decision making if they were consulting male doctors than if they were seeing female doctors and participated less than women patients consulting doctors of either gender, in this American study.

What information do people want?

People want 'real' information so that they know:

- ► what services are available, at practice or district levels, and how to access them
- ► how to make the best use of the services or facilities available
- ► what quality and quantity of services they are entitled to
- ► whether standards of care or service provision are being met
- ► what the options are for treating their condition – medical or social management, complementary or traditional therapy, invasive or conservative treatments or no treatment
- ► what the risks are for having, and not having, different treatments
- ► what the outcomes and side effects of treatment might be
- ► how to prevent a medical problem becoming worse, recurring or occurring in the first place
- ► what to expect whilst a treatment is being carried out and how they will feel
- ► what they can do to help themselves or the person they are caring for.

So if you review the standards of information being given to patients and the general public by the colleagues with whom you work, you will need to:

1 find out from patients what information they want – you cannot assume that those who provide healthcare know what information people require

2 identify subgroups of your patient or general public populations with particular information needs and think at the same time of the best ways to meet their needs. Would written or audio material suit them best or will it mean appointing someone to give out information personally face to face or via a telephone helpline?

3 review the quality of information patients are receiving; map out what is happening at present. Look to see how much of the literature or information available is out of date and if it is written or spoken at the right level for people's needs or understanding. Ask people if they found it useful and how the information might be improved

4 monitor that patients or the public receive the information that is available, especially hard-to-reach groups.

Informing the general public, including non-users of NHS services

Giving non-users information about services may make them more aware of how they might access healthcare, what is available and when it is appropriate for them to seek medical advice or help.

Informing the general public about health issues and the constraints on the NHS should enable them to share in decision making about allocating or rationing resources between competing services and between particular groups of people in the population. The open and accountable culture expected of the NHS includes sharing information with patients about costs and performance in the NHS. The increased emphasis on openness might encourage clinicians to become more candid too and tell patients what they really think about people who continue to gain weight, lie about having given up smoking or continue with a self-defeating lifestyle whilst taking antidepressant treatment!

Communicating information

Practices, PCGs and health authorities should be reviewing their communication strategies to provide the quality and quantity of information individuals or the public at large want. This will include:

► mapping out information requirements, including under-standing staff's and patients' different perspectives

► communication skills training for individual practitioners to improve their ability to involve patients in decision making about their own care, explain risks, give information at the right level for a particular patient's needs or understanding and determine their preferences

► structural changes to ensure that practitioners have ready access to electronic sources of reliable clinical information and guidelines, with the option of being able to print out associated patient information material (for example, the decision support programme, Prodigy). Medical libraries should be linked in

► direct access to reliable information for patients and the general public at large, for instance through practice-based libraries, telephone helplines or recommending particular Internet sites for lay people

► effective and appropriate information technology and computer skills training for all NHS staff

► the pooling of information relating to the determinants of health in respect of the local community held by the many health and social care organisations and local authority departments, so that practices, PCGs and health authorities have access to relevant socioeconomic and other health data for their populations

► improving the sharing of medical information about indi-vidual patients on a 'need-to-know' basis; this will include topics such as who has rights of personal and electronic access to medical records, shared care patient-held records, informed consent, confidentiality issues

► maintaining continuity of care and consistency of health messages with the increasing emphasis on multiprofessional working

► working with the media and press: briefing them proactively to get positive messages across and minimise negative or hostile reporting

► a steering group to oversee communication, for example with liaison groups to explain difficult issues at the interface between the NHS and media, or work with local communities; to co-ordinate the strategic objectives and work programme; and look after the dissemination of information to the target groups

► finding the resources to implement the communication strategy.

Telephone helplines

The three examples in the box show how hungry the general public is for basic information. Helplines could be a cost-effective option for practices, PCGs or health authorities to consider.

> **Telephone helplines – how popular are they and what information do they provide?**
>
> ► The district healthline in North Staffordshire takes on average 14 telephone calls per day from the general public. It is funded by the health authority and the Community Health Council. The service is staffed for six hours every weekday, with an answerphone for the rest of the time. A resource centre has been developed with literature and videos available to the public on loan. The most common information provided is about the availability of health services in the area (41% of callers) with 8% of callers wanting information about self-help and support groups, 2% about waiting times, 5% about Patient's Charter rights and
>
> *continued*

continued

standards, 6% advice about lifestyle and 18% information about diseases or medical conditions; 20% want advice on various other topics. The healthline staff welcome callers in person as well.

► A freephone national helpline for a hayfever treatment giving information about the day's pollen count attracted 55 000 calls in 1993.[6]

► A telephone helpline set up to give advice about arthritis after a television programme on the topic received 650 calls, mainly from women aged 50–70 years old.[7] Most wanted advice about pain control; concern about medication and side effects were common queries too.

Patient information leaflets

Leaflets are one way of providing patients with clear and easily understood information. Have a look at all the information leaflets in your cupboards at work and see if they:

► are easy to read, free of jargon and use straightforward text
► capture the reader's interest
► are relevant for: your setting, population, usual approach
► offer varied advice for: different age groups, reading ability, people with particular needs
► are up to date with information about evidence or best practice
► are accurate: messages are clear and not misleading
► give full details of all treatment alternatives, rather than being partisan and favouring a particular option (especially if supplied free from a commercial source)
► give balanced views about options, risks, side effects, uncertainties of investigation or treatment
► maintain a positive tone to encourage action and change behaviour for the better.

You could make your own leaflets: get your visiting physio-therapist or dietician to jot down their top tips and photocopy them. But it would be easier to use a standard electronic database from which you can print off your own leaflets. You can run copies off with the patient present and always be sure that patients are getting current literature, so long as your CD-ROM source is up to date. Some of the electronic packages that are available are given in Appendix 1.

The more interactive or visual the material you distribute to inform patients, the more likely it is to be successful in increasing the patient's understanding of the issue or the condition and engaging them in changing their behaviour. The kinds of ideas in circulation are:

▸ symptom diaries for patients to make regular records
▸ enrolling the patient on a register to receive regular mailings of information relating to a health condition or disease
▸ videos with associated information booklets for patients to log how their own symptoms and feelings compare
▸ pictorial representation of comparative risks of treatment
▸ checklists and quizzes to get patients relating the information to themselves or as screening tools looking for previously unrecognised health problems
▸ credit type cards for requesting priority appointments at the surgery (for example, given out in advance to adolescents in case they require emergency contraception or for people with severe mental health problems).

Patient's Charters

Patient's Charters may empower patients by publishing standards against which to measure the care and services that are available to them. But they cannot be successful if the published standards of care are unrealistic because of resource constraints and disappointed patients are frustrated by not receiving the care or services to which they were led to believe they were entitled. More could be made of the potential for charters to be used to publicise patients' responsibilities and help to control unnecessary demands on the NHS.

Communicating via the media

The local media are cheap and effective ways for practices, PCGs and health authorities to get information across to the local population. It is important for those working in the NHS to build up good relationships with individual editors, producers and journalists so that reports of successful initiatives and new developments are widely broadcast. You should be proactive and feed information to the media whilst the stories are current. The 'good' news will keep the local community informed and help to counterbalance the not-so-good articles and stories. There will be times when the developments planned by practices, PCGs and health authorities will be unpopular with the local community as care is shifted into the community or centralised to bigger hospitals, local units are closed and vulnerable people moved to live in community-based housing. If services are discontinued because of financial constraints or to make way for new services, the people who were receiving them may use a public protest to try to force continuation of the services. You should anticipate problems ahead and contact the media before the bad news breaks or the local community starts a campaign about unpopular decisions to discharge vulnerable people into the community. Brief the media with detailed information about the health issues or the funding constraints. Undertake pre-emptive work to explain about equality and that discrimination against particular subgroups of the population is unacceptable. Just as you should recognise the importance of involving lay people at an early stage in planning changes to NHS services, so you should engage with the media unless there are good reasons for regarding the information as being too sensitive for release into the public domain.

If you do speak on the radio, remember to be well prepared.

▶ Find out more about the programme and the person who will be interviewing you, whether it will be a straightforward interview or if the presenter usually tries to catch people out.

▶ Write down a few key points or 'sound bites' that you want to say at sometime in the interview.

▶ Write down the name of the presenter or other people involved so that you can use them.

▶ Use simple words, avoid jargon and speak clearly.

▶ Sit still and maintain the same distance from the microphone so that your voice sounds steady and confident.

▶ Write down any basic facts or statistics in case someone asks you; you might not remember in the heat of the moment.

▶ Try to sound friendly and relaxed and imagine you are just talking to a friend instead of a microphone.

▼

Make sure you have the basic facts at your fingertips if you agree to speak on the radio.

If you write an article for the local press:

▶ write in the usual style of the newspaper
▶ use simple words, short sentences and short paragraphs
▶ avoid jargon and complicated arguments
▶ give accurate information
▶ place your key points at the beginning of the paragraphs
▶ keep to the pre-agreed word count
▶ make an opening statement that will capture the reader's interest
▶ don't expect to be paid for the article necessarily, just be glad of the opportunity to get your views or messages across
▶ submit your article on time in line with the agreed deadline.

References

1 Kaplan SH, Greenfield S, Ware JE (1989) Assessing the effects of physician–patient interactions on the outcomes of chronic disease. *Med Care.* **33**(12): S110–27.

2 Hall JA, Roter DL, Katz NR (1988) Meta-analysis of correlates of provider behavior in medical encounters. *Med Care.* **26**(7): 657–75.

3 Which (1992) GPs, your verdict. *Which.* **April**: 202–5.

4 Grol R, Wensing M, Mainz J *et al.* (1999) Patients' priorities with respect to general practice care: an international comparison. *Fam Pract.* **16**(1): 4–11.

5 Kaplan SH, Gandek B, Greenfield S *et al.* (1995) Patients' and visit characteristics related to physicians' participatory decision-making style. *Med Care.* **33**(12): 1176–87.

6 Dyke P (1994) Freephone telephone numbers: what role will they play in patient/doctor information? *Med Dialogue.* **March**: 1–4.

7 Scott D (1994) Patient information: is this the way forward? *Med Dialogue.* **January**: 1–4.

Health information for health professionals, patients and the public

Useful organisations

Centre for Health Information Quality

The Centre acts as a source of expertise and knowledge for the NHS and patient representative groups on all aspects of patient information, to improve the NHS's capability, competence and capacity to provide good, evidence-based patient information.

Contact: Centre for Health Information Quality, Highcroft, Romsey Road, Winchester, SO22 5DH. Tel: 01962 863511 ext 200. Fax: 01962 840454.

College of Health

The College of Health is a national charity founded to represent the interests of patients. The College publishes a range of reports, guidelines and packs based on independent research.

Contact: Publications Unit, College of Health, St Margaret's House, 21 Old Ford Road, London E2 9PL. Tel: 0181 983 1225. Fax: 0181 983 1553.

Consumer Health Information Consortium

CHIC is a support organisation which provides training, encourages good practice and promotes free, open access to health information for all. It acts as a network for individuals or organisations concerned with consumer health information. *Contact*: Chair, CHIC, c/o Hospital Library, St Thomas' Hospital, North Wing, London SE1 7EH. Tel: 0171 928 9292 ext 2507. Fax: 0171 922 8251.

Health Promotion Information Centre
The Centre has a series of health-related databases for health professionals on specific population groups: young people, older people, black and minority ethnic groups and people with learning disabilities. The databases include up-to-date information about nationally available resources that promote health and healthy living. The databases can be accessed via http:/healthpromis.hea.org.uk or a search can be requested through HPIC. Tel: 0171 413 1995. Fax: 0171 413 2605. Email: hpic.enquiry@hea.org.uk

Help for Health Trust
The Trust aims to provide people with the information they need to make healthy choices. It provides a freephone health information service (0800 665544) for patients and carers in central/southern England, produces databases of consumer health information and has a specialist health information research unit.
Contact: Help for Health Trust, Highcroft, Romsey Road, Winchester, SO22 5DH. Tel: 01962 841100. Fax: 01962 849079.

King's Fund
The King's Fund is an independent health charity that promotes the health of people in London through policy analysis and development and information about health and social care. It has five major programmes of policy and development work: community care, effective practice, health systems, primary care and public health, and key themes include promoting cultural diversity, tackling health inequalities and developing public involvement.
Contact: King's Fund, 11–13 Cavendish Square, London W1M 0AN. Tel: 0171 307 2668/9.
Website: www.kingsfund.org.uk

NHS Centre for Reviews and Dissemination (CRD)
The Centre provides the NHS with information on the effectiveness and cost-effectiveness of treatments and the delivery
and organisation of healthcare. It aims to disseminate research
to the medical profession, nurses, midwives, health visitors
and professions allied to medicine (PAMS).
Contact: NHS Centre for Reviews and Dissemination, University of York, York, YO1 5DD. Tel: 01904 433634 (general
enquiries), 01904 433707 (information service), 01904 433648
(publications).

Royal College of General Practitioners
College publications and other patient-centred literature are
available from the Sales Office.
Contact: Sales Office, Royal College of General Practitioners,
14 Princes Gate, Hyde Park, London SW7 1PU. Tel: 0171
823 9698. Fax: 0171 225 0629. Email: sales@rcgp.org.uk

Scottish Association of Health Councils
18 Alva Street, Edinburgh EH2 4QG.

Useful material for patients, managers and health professionals

**Ask the Patient series, User Involvement, Consumer
Audit, Primary Health Care, Rationing, Disabled
People:** many reports and guidelines in these topics published
by the College of Health (see above for contact details).

**Coulter A, Entwistle V, Gilbert D (1998) Informing
Patients: An Assessment of the Quality of Patient
Information Materials**, King's Fund, ISBN 185717 214 0.
Much existing patient information material is out of date,
inaccurate and misleading. The book demonstrates how the
NHS can improve material to help patients share in decision

making about their treatments from an informed standpoint (see above for contact details).

Department of Health catalogue of free publications and information

The catalogue aims to provide an up-to-date index of all publicity material in an easy-to-follow guide. To order the catalogue and free publications write to: Department of Health, PO Box 410, Wetherby, LS23 7EN or fax 0990 210 266.

eMIMS

This CD-ROM is a prescribing information package designed for GPs. It includes pictures of every tablet or capsule, patient information leaflets, prescribing notes on diseases and videos. *Contact*: Haymarket Medical Limited, 174 Hammersmith Road, London W6 7JP. Tel: 0181 267 4681. Fax: 0181 267 4878. Email: emims@haynet.com

Gaskin K (1997) How to Work with Your Doctor Royal College of General Practitioners, London (see above for contact details).

Help is a comprehensive guide to over 800 British self-help groups and support organisations.
Contact: G-Text, Freepost NWW6775, Blackpool, FY4 3GA. Email: g-text@blackpool.net

Kelson M (1998) Promoting Patient Involvement in Clinical Audit College of Health (see above for contact details).

McIver S (1993) Obtaining the Views of Health Service Users about the Quality of Information King's Fund, London (see above for contact details).

Olszewski D, Jones L (1998) Putting People in the Picture Scottish Association of Health Councils, Edinburgh (see above for contact details).

Patient Pictures
Range of books containing clinical drawings for use by doctors and nurses when describing medical conditions and treatments to their patients, covering basic anatomy, disease progress, investigations and treatments. Available from the Sales Office, Royal College of General Practitioners (see above for contact details).

PhysioTools
Produce CDs for GPs to make their own patient information leaflets on home care for stroke patients and incontinence.
Contact: PIP Professionals on 01749 890870. Website: www.physiotools.com

RTFB Publishing
Provide customised patient education materials for health authorities and PCGs, including booklets, leaflets and audio cassettes.
Contact: RTFB Publishing Ltd, Building 2, Shamrock Quay, Southampton, SO14 5QL. Tel: 01703 229041. Fax: 01703 227274.

Useful British websites

AIDS/HIV : Terrence Higgins Trust
http://www.tht.org.uk/

Alzheimer's Disease Society
http://www.alzheimers.org.uk

Arthritis and Rheumatism Council
http://rheuma.bham.ac.uk/arc.html

Asthma and Allergy Research
http://www.users.globalnet.co.uk/~aair/

BACUP
http://medweb.bham.ac.uk/cancerhelp/public/bacup/

British Digestive Foundation
http://www.bdf.org.uk/

Deaf and Hard of Hearing
http://web.ukonline.co.uk/hearing.concern/

Dental phobics information
http://www.dentalfear.org/

Diabetes: adults
http://www.diabetic.org.uk/index/htm

Disabled Living Foundation
http://www.atlas.co.uk/dlf/

Epilepsy
http://www.epilepsy.org.uk/

Hepatitis Network
http://www.hepnet.com/

Institute of Psychiatry
http://www.iop.bpmf.ac.uk/

Marie Stopes Institute
http://www.mariestopes.org.uk/

Mental Health Foundation
http://www.mentalhealth.org.uk/

Multiple sclerosis
http://www.mssociety.org.uk/

Prostate Help Association
http://www.u-net.com/~pha/

Spina bifida and hydrocephalus
http://www.asbah.demon.co.uk/ifhsb.html

The Voluntary Organisations Internet Server
http://www.vois.org.uk/newhtml/about.html

Training and Awareness Programme in Networks
http://www.bham.ac.uk/tapin/medicine.htm

Twins and Multiple Births Association
http://www.surreyweb.org.uk/tamba/

Women's health: infertility
http://ferti.net/uk/index.htm

Media – useful contacts

Association of Broadcasting Doctors
Publishes a regular newsletter updating members about advances in medicine and news of the profession, about which they might broadcast or write.
Contact: Peter Petts, Association of Broadcasting Doctors, Freepost, PO Box 15, Ely, Cambridge CB7 4BR. Tel: 01353 688 456/588. Fax: 01353 688451. Email: Soundplan@dial.pipex.com

General Practitioner Writers Association
Has a regular journal and database of authors with areas of interest and expertise. Editors commission articles from the database. GPs, health professionals and others with an interest in health may join as members. Has twice-yearly residential meetings and a regular newsletter.
Contact: The General Secretary, GPWA, 633 Liverpool Road, Southport, Merseyside PR8 3NG. Tel: 01704 577839.

Media Medics
Gives regular updates on current clinical topics to enable members to give advice on the subject on the radio. Circulates members with other items of interest that might be newsworthy. Occasional national meeting.
Contact: Claybrooke, Haywards, Pound Hill, Crawley, Sussex RH10 3TR. Tel: 01293 889100. Fax: 01293 882100.

Media Workshop
Offers intensive, structured one and two-day courses in communication skills for speaking in public or dealing with the media.

Contact: Anna Jackson, Media Workshop, 44 Thornton Avenue, London W4 1QG. Tel: 0181 995 6140.

Tim Albert Training to Improve Your Writing Skills
One-day public courses on effective writing, writing scientific papers and setting up newsletters. Run courses in London or for inhouse groups elsewhere.
Contact: Paper Mews Court, 284 High Street, Dorking, Surrey RH4 1QT. Tel: 01306 877993. Email: tatraining@ compuserve.com

► APPENDIX 2

The General Practice Assessment Survey

This is reproduced with the kind permission of the National Primary Care Research and Development Centre (NPCRDC), University of Manchester, www.npcrdc.man.ac.uk

The GPAS measures access and availability, technical care, interpersonal care (including listening, explaining, time, caring and patience), continuity of care, trust, contextual knowledge (how well the doctor knows the patient), practice nursing care, referral and co-ordination of care outside the practice. You do not need permission to use the GPAS questionnaire. You can photocopy it and use it without charge. The NPCRDC and the Health Institute must be acknowledged using the form of words at the bottom of the first page of the printed questionnaire.

The scoring system should be obtained from the associated manual produced by the NPCRDC (*see* website).

You and Your Doctor

The General Practice
Assessment Survey (GPAS)

1 How **long** have you been registered with your practice?

- ❏ 1 **Less than 1 year**
- ❏ 2 **1 to 2 years**
- ❏ 3 **3 to 4 years**
- ❏ 4 **More than 4 years**

2 In the **past 12 months**, how many times have you seen a doctor or a nurse from your practice?

- ❏ 1 **None**
- ❏ 2 **Once or twice**
- ❏ 3 **Three or four times**
- ❏ 4 **Five times or more**

3 How would you rate the convenience of your practice's **location?**

- ❏ 1 **Very poor**
- ❏ 2 **Poor**
- ❏ 3 **Fair**
- ❏ 4 **Good**
- ❏ 5 **Very good**
- ❏ 6 **Excellent**

4 How would you rate the way you are treated by the **receptionists** in your practice?

- ❏ 1 **Very poor**
- ❏ 2 **Poor**
- ❏ 3 **Fair**
- ❏ 4 **Good**
- ❏ 5 **Very good**
- ❏ 6 **Excellent**

5 a How would you rate the **hours** that your practice is open for appointments?

- ❏ 1 **Very poor**
- ❏ 2 **Poor**
- ❏ 3 **Fair**
- ❏ 4 **Good**
- ❏ 5 **Very good**
- ❏ 6 **Excellent**

b What **additional** hours would you like your practice to be open? (Please tick all that apply)

- ❏ 1 **Early morning**
- ❏ 2 **Evenings**
- ❏ 3 **Weekends**
- ❏ 4 **None, I am satisfied**

6   Thinking of times when you want to see a **particular** doctor:
     a How quickly do you get an appointment?

❑ 1   ❑ 2   ❑ 3   ❑ 4   ❑ 5   ❑ 6
Same   **Next**   **2–3**   **4–5**   **More than**   **Does**
day   **day**   **days**   **days**   **5 days**   **not apply**

     b How do you rate this?

❑ 1   ❑ 2   ❑ 3   ❑ 4   ❑ 5   ❑ 6   ❑ 7
Very **Poor** **Fair** **Good** **Very**   **Excellent** **Does not**
poor   **good**   **apply**

---

7   Thinking of times when you are willing to see **any** doctor:
     a How quickly do you get an appointment?

❑ 1   ❑ 2   ❑ 3   ❑ 4   ❑ 5   ❑ 6
Same   **Next**   **2–3**   **4–5**   **More than**   **Does**
day   **day**   **days**   **days**   **5 days**   **not apply**

     b How do you rate this?

❑ 1   ❑ 2   ❑ 3   ❑ 4   ❑ 5   ❑ 6   ❑ 7
Very **Poor** **Fair** **Good** **Very**   **Excellent** **Does not**
poor   **good**   **apply**

---

8   If you need an urgent appointment to see your GP can you
     normally get one on the same day?
     Yes ❑ 1   **No** ❑ 2   **Don't know/never needed one** ❑ 3

---

9   a How long do you have to wait at the practice for your
       appointments to begin?

❑ 1   **Not at all, they begin on time**
❑ 2   **Less than 5 minutes**
❑ 3   **6 to 10 minutes**
❑ 4   **11 to 20 minutes**
❑ 5   **21 to 30 minutes**
❑ 6   **31 to 45 minutes**
❑ 7   **More than 45 minutes**

     b How do you rate this?

❑ 1   ❑ 2   ❑ 3   ❑ 4   ❑ 5   ❑ 6
Very **Poor** **Fair** **Good** **Very**   **Excellent**
poor   **good**

10 Thinking about the times you have phoned the practice, how would you rate the following?

a Ability to **get through to** the practice on the phone.

❑ 1	❑ 2	❑ 3	❑ 4	❑ 5	❑ 6	❑ 7
Very poor	**Poor**	**Fair**	**Good**	**Very good**	**Excellent**	**Don't know**

b Ability to **speak to** a doctor on the phone when you have a question or need medical advice.

❑ 1	❑ 2	❑ 3	❑ 4	❑ 5	❑ 6	❑ 7
Very poor	**Poor**	**Fair**	**Good**	**Very good**	**Excellent**	**Don't know**

11 a In general, how often do you see your usual doctor (not an assistant or partner)?

❑ 1	❑ 2	❑ 3	❑ 4	❑ 5	❑ 6
Always	**Almost always**	**A lot of the time**	**Some of the time**	**Almost never**	**Never**

b How do you rate this?

❑ 1	❑ 2	❑ 3	❑ 4	❑ 5	❑ 6
Very poor	**Poor**	**Fair**	**Good**	**Very good**	**Excellent**

12 **The next questions ask you about your *usual doctor*. If you don't identify one doctor as your usual doctor answer the questions about the doctor in the practice who you feel you know best. If you don't know any of the doctors, go straight to Question 25.**

13 Thinking about the **technical aspects** of your care, how would you rate the following:

a Your doctor's **medical knowledge**.

❏ 1   ❏ 2   ❏ 3   ❏ 4   ❏ 5   ❏ 6   ❏ 7

Very poor   **Poor**   **Fair**   **Good**   **Very good**   **Excellent**   **Don't know**

b Thoroughness of doctor's **physical examination** of you to check a health problem.

❏ 1   ❏ 2   ❏ 3   ❏ 4   ❏ 5   ❏ 6   ❏ 7

Very poor   **Poor**   **Fair**   **Good**   **Very good**   **Excellent**   **Don't know**

c Arranging the **tests** you need when you are unwell (e.g. blood tests, x-rays, etc).

❏ 1   ❏ 2   ❏ 3   ❏ 4   ❏ 5   ❏ 6   ❏ 7

Very poor   **Poor**   **Fair**   **Good**   **Very good**   **Excellent**   **Don't know**

d Prescribing the right **treatment** for you.

❏ 1   ❏ 2   ❏ 3   ❏ 4   ❏ 5   ❏ 6   ❏ 7

Very poor   **Poor**   **Fair**   **Good**   **Very good**   **Excellent**   **Don't know**

e Making the right **diagnosis**.

❏ 1   ❏ 2   ❏ 3   ❏ 4   ❏ 5   ❏ 6   ❏ 7

Very poor   **Poor**   **Fair**   **Good**   **Very good**   **Excellent**   **Don't know**

14 Thinking about **talking** with your usual doctor, how would you rate the following:

a Thoroughness of your doctor's **questions** about your symptoms and how you are feeling.

❏ 1   ❏ 2   ❏ 3   ❏ 4   ❏ 5   ❏ 6

Very poor   **Poor**   **Fair**   **Good**   **Very good**   **Excellent**

b Attention the doctor gives to what you say.

❏ 1   ❏ 2   ❏ 3   ❏ 4   ❏ 5   ❏ 6

Very poor   **Poor**   **Fair**   **Good**   **Very good**   **Excellent**

c Doctor's **explanations** of your health problems or treatments that you need.

❏ 1   ❏ 2   ❏ 3   ❏ 4   ❏ 5   ❏ 6

Very good   **Poor**   **Fair**   **Good**   **Very good**   **Excellent**

15 How often do you leave your doctor's surgery with **unanswered questions?**

❏¹   ❏²   ❏³   ❏⁴   ❏⁵   ❏⁶
Always   **Almost**   **A lot**   **Some**   **Almost**   **Never**
               always   **of the**   **of the**   **never**
                                             time   **time**

16 Thinking about the **personal aspects** of the care that you receive from your usual doctor, how would you rate the following:

a Amount of **time** your doctor spends with you.

❏¹   ❏²   ❏³   ❏⁴   ❏⁵   ❏⁶
Very poor **Poor**   **Fair**   **Good**   **Very good**   **Excellent**

b Doctor's **patience** with your questions or worries.

❏¹   ❏²   ❏³   ❏⁴   ❏⁵   ❏⁶
Very poor **Poor**   **Fair**   **Good**   **Very good**   **Excellent**

c Doctor's **caring and concern** for you.

❏¹   ❏²   ❏³   ❏⁴   ❏⁵   ❏⁶
Very poor **Poor**   **Fair**   **Good**   **Very good**   **Excellent**

17 Thinking about how much you **trust** your doctor, how strongly do you *agree* or *disagree* with the following statements:

a I completely trust my doctor's **judgements** about my medical care.

❏¹   ❏²   ❏³   ❏⁴   ❏⁵
Strongly   **Agree**   **Not sure**   **Disagree**   **Strongly**
agree   **disagree**

b My doctor would always tell me the **truth** about my health, even if there was bad news.

❏¹   ❏²   ❏³   ❏⁴   ❏⁵
Strongly   **Agree**   **Not sure**   **Disagree**   **Strongly**
agree   **disagree**

c My doctor cares more about **keeping down** costs than about doing what is needed for my health.

❏¹   ❏²   ❏³   ❏⁴   ❏⁵
Strongly   **Agree**   **Not sure**   **Disagree**   **Strongly**
agree   **disagree**

18   All things considered, how much do you **trust** your doctor?
     (Please tick one number)

     ❏   ❏   ❏   ❏   ❏   ❏   ❏   ❏   ❏   ❏
     1   2   3   4   5   6   7   8   9   10
Not at all   **Completely**

---

19   Thinking about how well your doctor **knows you**, how would
     you rate the following:
     a Doctor's knowledge of your **medical history**.

     ❏ 1   ❏ 2   ❏ 3   ❏ 4   ❏ 5   ❏ 6
     Very poor   **Poor**   **Fair**   **Good**   **Very good**   **Excellent**

     b Doctor's knowledge of what **worries** you most about your
        health.

     ❏ 1   ❏ 2   ❏ 3   ❏ 4   ❏ 5   ❏ 6
     Very poor   **Poor**   **Fair**   **Good**   **Very good**   **Excellent**

     c Doctor's knowledge of your **responsibilities** at home, work or
        school.

     ❏ 1   ❏ 2   ❏ 3   ❏ 4   ❏ 5   ❏ 6
     Very poor   **Poor**   **Fair**   **Good**   **Very good**   **Excellent**

---

20   Have you seen a **nurse** in your practice in the last year?
     Yes ❏ 1   **No** ❏ 2
If **Yes** please go to **Question 21**.
If **No** please go to **Question 22**.

21 Thinking about the nurses you have seen, how would you rate the following:

a The **attention** they give to what you say.

❏ 1   ❏ 2   ❏ 3   ❏ 4   ❏ 5   ❏ 6

Very poor   Poor   Fair   Good   Very good   Excellent

b The **quality** of care they provide.

❏ 1   ❏ 2   ❏ 3   ❏ 4   ❏ 5   ❏ 6

Very poor   Poor   Fair   Good   Very good   Excellent

c Their **explanations** of your health problems or treatments that you need.

❏ 1   ❏ 2   ❏ 3   ❏ 4   ❏ 5   ❏ 6

Very poor   Poor   Fair   Good   Very good   Excellent

---

22 Thinking about the last 12 months, was there any time when your doctor didn't send you to a **specialist** when you thought you needed it?

Yes ❏ 1   **No** ❏ 2

---

23 Does your doctor **co-ordinate** care that you receive from outside the practice?

❏ 1   ❏ 2   ❏ 3   ❏ 4

Yes a lot   Yes a little   Not at all   Does not apply

---

24 Would you **recommend** your usual doctor to your family and friends?

❏ 1   ❏ 2   ❏ 3   ❏ 4   ❏ 5

Definitely not   Probably not   Not sure   Probably yes   Definitely yes

25 All things considered, how **satisfied** are you with your practice?
- ❏ ¹   **Completely satisfied, couldn't be better**
- ❏ ²   **Very satisfied**
- ❏ ³   **Somewhat satisfied**
- ❏ ⁴   **Neither satisfied nor dissatisfied**
- ❏ ⁵   **Somewhat dissatisfied**
- ❏ ⁶   **Very dissatisfied**
- ❏ ⁷   **Completely dissatisfied, couldn't be worse**

26 Are you: ❏ ¹ Male   ❏ ² Female

27 What is your date of birth?   Day   Month   Year

          _____   _____   _____

28 Are you:
❏ ¹ **Single**   ❏ ² **Married/cohabiting**   ❏ ³ **Widow/er, divorced or separated**

29 To which of these groups do you consider you belong? (Please tick one box only)

White	❏ ¹
Black – Caribbean	❏ ²
Black – African	❏ ³
Black – Other	❏ ⁴ Please describe
Indian	❏ ⁵
Pakistani	❏ ⁶
Bangladeshi	❏ ⁷
Chinese	❏ ⁸
Any other ethnic group	❏ ⁹ Please describe

30 Do you have any **long-standing illness, disability or infirmity**? By long-standing I mean anything that has troubled you over a period of time or that is likely to affect you over a period of time.

Yes ❏ ¹   **No** ❏ ²

31 How is your health in general? Would you say it is:
❑¹ ❑² ❑³ ❑⁴ ❑⁵
Very good **Good** **Fair** **Bad** **Very bad**

32 Is your accommodation:
❑¹ **Owner-occupied?**
❑² **Rented from local authority/housing association?**
❑³ **Rented from a private landlord?**
❑⁴ **Or is it under other arrangements?**
If so, please describe:

33 Is there a **car or van** normally available for use by you?
Yes ❑¹   **No** ❑²
If yes, how many are normally available?
One ❑¹   **Two or more** ❑²

Acknowledgement: the following items in the GPAS have been adapted, with permission, from the Primary Care Assessment Survey (PCAS), © 1996 Safran/The Health Institute: Items 1–3, 5–7, 9–11, 13b, 14–19, 24–25.

Patient Enablement Instrument

The Patient Enablement Instrument has been developed in the Department of General Practice in Edinburgh. It is still undergoing further research and its use has not yet been shown to improve quality of care. The questionnaire is reproduced here by kind permission of Professor Howie. You may use it without further permission. Further guidance on the use of the questionnaire is available from Professor John Howie, Department of General Practice, Levinson House, 20 West Richmond Street, Edinburgh EH8 9DX. The method of scoring is given in: Howie JGR, Heaney D, Maxwell M, Walker JJ (1998) A comparison of the Patient Enablement Instrument (PEI) against two established satisfaction scales as an outcome measure of primary care consultations. *Fam Pract.* **15**: 165–71.

As a result of your visit to the doctor, do you feel that you are:	Much Better	Better	Same or Less	Not Applicable
able to cope with life	❏	❏	❏	❏
able to understand your your illness	❏	❏	❏	❏
able to cope with your illness	❏	❏	❏	❏
able to keep yourself healthy	❏	❏	❏	❏
confident about your health	❏	❏	❏	❏
able to help yourself	❏	❏	❏	❏

▶ INDEX